MODERN
HOME REMEDIES
and How to Use Them

MODERN
HOME
REMEDIES

and

How to Use Them

MORRIS FISHBEIN, M.D.

DOUBLEDAY & COMPANY, INC.   1966   NEW YORK

CONTENTS

PREFACE

The food and drug laws of the United States make a distinction between the drugs which a person may buy without a prescription and those which the doctor must prescribe. Both types are likely on occasion to carry on the labels required warnings of possible harmful effects.

Many common afflictions are so ephemeral or insignificant that people are accustomed to attempt to control the symptoms without recourse to the doctor. Such self-treatment is facilitated by the fact that many preparations contain on their labels full lists of the ingredients. Some of these are simply flavoring or solvents, one or two at most being principal or potent ingredients. These are highly standardized. Practically all pain relievers contain aspirin. Laxatives may contain cascara, senna, salts, phenolphthalein, or similar well-known substances.

A British publication called "Ailments and Remedies" recently printed a list of "do's and don'ts" of self-medication. I have selected a few particularly applicable to American readers:

1. Read the label and follow the instructions.

2. Do not take any drugs during the early months of pregnancy unless the doctor is informed about them and recommends their use.

7

3. If the symptoms do not begin to improve after a reasonable time, consult your doctor.

4. If a new symptom develops while you are taking any drug preparation, tell the doctor. This applies particularly to nausea, dizziness, eruptions of the skin, or vomiting.

5. Keep all preparations out of the reach of children.

MORRIS FISHBEIN, M.D.

Chicago
January 31, 1966

One
WHY SELF-MEDICATION?

In the United States pharmacies are permitted to sell over-the-counter remedies which are safe when taken according to the directions. More powerful and specific remedies must be prescribed by a doctor. People should not, of course, attempt to treat themselves for any serious condition. However, minor symptoms are often easily cared for.

Before 1900 physicians were doubtful about anyone attempting to treat himself. The tradition that prevailed then was that all remedies were unsafe except when prescribed by a doctor. Doctors in those days disapproved of the patient taking a laxative or cathartic, a tablet for a cold, a syrup for a cough, or anything that might be rubbed on the skin. Scientific pharmacy had not yet developed the antiseptics that destroy germs, the treatments for itching, the drugs that stop congestion in the nose, or any of the modern drugs that can reduce pain or induce sleep.

Today all that is changed.

The Council on Pharmacy and Chemistry of the American Medical Association long since recognized the desirability of having so-called "household remedies" available to the general public. In the many years that have passed, I know of few instances when over-the-counter remedies have had an adverse effect on the purchaser. In England "household remedies" are available on the open shelves in all of the drugstores or chemists' shops and on the open shelves of department stores. I know of no laws in England that will prevent their sales in supermarkets when England has them. In Italy one may purchase anti-sea- and air-sickness remedies "over the counter" and in some places on open self-service shelves. Airplane hostesses dispense aspirin, Dramamine, and similar remedies. After flying more than a million miles I have never seen harm result from such administration. The United States Army dispenses millions of doses of relief-giving agents for this condition, in most instances leaving the dispensing to non-medical officers or even enlisted men. The formula used by the Army is available in many proprietary preparations. I doubt that either a pharmacist or a physician is needed to dispense these.

Headache remedies are a good example of medications which virtually must be made available to the public. The vast majority of headaches may be due to emotional stress, slight variations in the circulation of the blood, or hundreds of other minor causes. Relief is easily accomplished with many available proprietary remedies. It would be simply impossible for physicians to see all the people who have headaches at the time when they have the headaches. As for choosing a remedy, I doubt that any licensed pharmacist is better able to decide than the person who has tried a half dozen remedies and has found one that helps him. Of course persistent headaches require a medical diagnosis.

Nausea related to dietary indiscretions is another proper area for self-treatment, but with a qualification. The 15–20 per cent of the American people who suffer with symptoms of excessive stomach acidity and who are accustomed to treating themselves with baking soda (sodium bicarbonate) or with any of several dozen innocuous substances that lessen irritation, should actually have diagnoses to identify the condition correctly. Once the condition is recognized, little necessity exists for either the physician or pharmacist to prescribe every time it needs alleviation.

Today there are a steadily increasing number of safe over-the-counter medicines for a wide range of minor ailments. There are many remedies for itching conceded to be relatively, if not absolutely, harmless. Insect bites, poison ivy, poison oak, occasional sensitivities to food, all demand easy access to quick remedies. Persistent symptoms should always lead to consultation with doctors or pharmacists.

Our existing federal and state laws afford a maximum of protection in this country compared with most other countries where I have traveled. Over the years it has become apparent that any substance used to excess may be harmful, including water. Therefore, restrictions have been placed on substances likely to be used in excess. But sale of aspirin, cough drops, headache remedies, substances for the relief of colds, milk of magnesia and other laxatives without intermediation which would add to the costs is permitted. Restrictions which would make access to these substances more difficult would, I am sure, be opposed by the public.

Among the most frequent users of home remedies and products purchased over the counter are the aged, of whom there are now about eighteen million in the United States. The cost of medical care of these people is a cause for concern. More than a few competent geriatricians (specialists in care of the aged) are convinced that old people need a regular intake of certain vitamins. This is because, first, they do not eat well, second, they do not absorb well what they eat, and third, they frequently suffer with symptoms indicating that they need the vitamins whose absence is associated with certain effects. I have in mind particularly the vitamins of the B complex, some of which are said to enhance appetite and indeed to improve alertness. Some in the B complex are related to digestion, and one vitamin is concerned with the production of red blood cells. Old people are particularly unlikely to have sufficient calcium and with it the vitamins concerned with proper absorption and utilization of calcium. Old people suffer inordinately with dizziness, with itching, and with a number of other discomforts

which are in most instances easily relieved by certain
home remedies. Few physicians would not agree that
such patients be instructed as to what they should have
and what they should purchase regularly in sufficient
quantities to meet their needs.

DO'S AND DON'TS FOR
HOME REMEDIES

Home remedies should be used only for minor ailments
of short duration. If unusual symptoms such as rapid
pulse, dizziness, or blurring of vision occur, the medicine
should be discontinued. If pain persists for more than ten
days or if there is redness and swelling, a physician should
be consulted immediately.

Here are some simple rules from a pamphlet published
by The Food and Drug Administration of the Department
of Health, Education, and Welfare:

1. Date all over-the-counter drugs when you
buy them. Prescription drugs will be dated by the
pharmacist.

2. Buy medicines and health supplies in realistic
quantities. Old drugs deteriorate and may become ineffective or even dangerous.

3. Be sure to store all drugs out of the way of small
children, under lock and key if they cannot be protected any other way.

4. Safeguard particularly tablets which are candied, flavored, or colored, since small children eat them like candy.

5. Never give or take medicine from an unlabeled bottle. Transparent tape over the label will protect it.

6. Never take or give medicine in the dark. Be sure the label can be read clearly.

7. Before measuring liquid medicine, always shake the bottle thoroughly.

8. When measuring drugs, give the job full attention.

9. Weed out the leftovers regularly from the home medicine chest—especially any prescription drugs that may have been ordered for a prior illness.

10. When you throw away drugs, flush them down the toilet, and be sure the discarded containers cannot be reached by children or pets.

GRASSROOTS MEDICINE AND FOLKLORE

The fact that medicine is not an exclusive preserve of doctors is nothing new. Ordinary people devoid of medical training or knowledge have been treating themselves for centuries. Sometimes they have done so with amazingly good effect.

Many of the most important discoveries in medicine and particularly in the treatment of disease have been made through accidental use by people not medically trained. The use of sulphur for the treatment of seven-year itch was developed by an old Italian market woman. The use of digitalis for eliminating fluids from the body was discovered by a woman herb doctor in England. The American Indians discovered the value of leaves of wintergreen for rheumatic aches and pains; later scientists found that wintergreen contains methylsalicylate, which is used for lowering fevers as well as for rheumatic pains. The Indians also discovered the purgative action of the bark of cascara. The Incas of Peru discovered the fatigue-relieving properties of coca leaves. The natives of the Amazon found curare, which they used for a poison but which is today an ingredient of antispasmodic drugs. The Incas also discovered the sweat-producing properties of ipecac, and found out that it can cause vomiting. The Moslems discovered the stimulating and awakening powers of coffee, which contains caffeine, and the fatigue-relieving properties of tea, which contains theobromine. Many different peoples found that fruit juices or grain mashes fermented when exposed to warmth and sunlight, from which came the innumerable alcoholic drinks also used in medicines. In Peru cinchona bark was found to have value in malaria.

Many home medical practices have come down from rural people without access to medication. Some of these practices lack any scientific basis; others have actual physiological effects. Some, too, have psychological effects. Rheumatic pains, for example, are often as much psychological as actual, and copper pennies in the shoes, rings made out of horseshoe nails, buckeye seeds in the hip pocket, may have had therapeutic value. The American Indians used decoctions of willow bark for aches and pains. This contains considerable amounts of salicylates, as do also cranberries. For conditions affecting the lungs, many rural people have used inhalations of hot steam and smoke. For asthma a wide variety of smokes has been tried, none having any real scientific merit. Hot lemonade has been used for years to ward off colds but without any proof that it really does so. Purgatives of all kinds have been used, including heroic doses of salts.

In Arkansas and New Hampshire rural people have treated diarrhea with blackberry root and juice. In Arkansas smartweed and teas made from sassafras bark and other weeds have been used for the same purpose. For many years bread-and-milk poultices have been applied to inflammations and wounds. It has been suggested that such poultices may have had some antibiotic effect, since penicillin and other antibiotics derive from bread and other moulds. In rural America many years ago spring tonics were regularly employed, consisting usually of any herb, weed, or chemical that had a suitably bitter taste. The value of these tonics or "blood medicines" is dubious.

HOME MEDICATION GROWS UP

Today self-treatment at home is on a level of medical sophistication our grandmothers would hardly have suspected. In the first place, people are far better educated medically than was the case a generation or two ago. Health information has been widely disseminated through newspapers, magazines, and books. These well-informed people then have the benefit of an enormous wealth of packaged remedies and treatments for minor ailments which carry built-in safeguards in their strictly controlled testing and labeling. Drugs sold over the counter are considered misbranded if their claims are false or misleading, or if they carry inadequate warnings against misuse, or even if they do not specify dosages for adults and for children.

ASPIRIN—THE HOME-REMEDY KING

Of the $1.5 billion spent annually in the United States on non-prescription drugs, the biggest single share goes to buy aspirin, of which some one thousand different preparations are available to the public. It may come as plain aspirin, effervescent preparations, mixtures of aspirin and salicylates, long-acting aspirin, and mixtures of aspirin with other drugs. There are also flavored aspirin preparations for children.

Dr. Arthur Grollmann of the Department of Experimental Medicine of the University of Texas says that the analgesics (pain relievers) and antipyretics (which reduce fever) are the most widely used of all medications. Aspirin and other pain relievers are used for headache, arthritic pains, and for the general ill feelings that are associated with most infectious diseases. Aspirin has an anti-inflammatory effect and is, therefore, used also for rheumatic inflammations. One reason why aspirin is used so widely and successfully is that it is absorbed rapidly not only from the stomach but also from the small intestine. Usually it is circulating at its peak in the blood within two hours. Its clinical effectiveness lasts about three hours. Therefore people renew the dose about every three hours.

Many other varieties of salicylic acid are used in pain relievers. The classic formula of aspirin, phenacetin, and caffeine makes a remedy that became widely known during World War II as APC. The caffeine was used as a stimulant, and phenacetin is believed to enhance the action of the aspirin so that smaller doses of both may be used when combined.

THE ANTACIDS

Among the drugs most used for gastrointestinal conditions are antacids which act against excess acid in the stomach. Most often the acidity of the gastric contents rises after a meal and then declines rapidly. In some conditions, however, the acidity may remain high for many hours, accompanied by pain, cramping, and belching. When the excess acid is neutralized, the symptoms are relieved. Many antacids are available and can be purchased over the counter. Baking soda is often used but acts for only a short time. There are also hydroxides, oxides, silicates, carbonates, and phosphates of calcium, magnesium, bismuth, and aluminum. Aluminum hydroxide is also used for diarrheas. Magnesium hydroxide and magnesium trisilicate are palatable and therefore widely used. Manufacturers have developed many products of this kind which are sold under trade names in drugstores.

LAXATIVES

Constipation is probably the most common complaint of civilized man. It may result from a great variety of causes but is usually due to the failure of the bowel to react properly to the presence of the mass of waste material. When failure to respond to an urge becomes habitual, the condition becomes chronic. The home remedies used for constipation include milk of magnesia, mineral oil, cascara, and other vegetable preparations, salts, and phenolphthalein. Still widely used are older cathartics such as castor oil, sulphur, and senna preparations. Rarely used now is calomel. Some of these preparations act by irritating the bowel, some by causing water to flow into the bowel, and some by stimulating the nerve connections in the bowel. When these drugs are used properly, little harm results. However, continuous use may result in overstimulation of the bowel so that it becomes even more insensitive.

Other home remedies are used for dyspepsia, indigestion, nausea, lack of appetite, and diarrhea. Still more recently in connection with overweight, preparations have become available to decrease the appetite. Some remedies are used to aid digestion. These usually contain enzymes like papain or bile salts and pancreatin. Bile is important in the digestion of fats.

IRON PREPARATIONS

A condition found frequently in American young people and old people is anemia. Usually it is a secondary anemia, which can be treated effectively with iron. Iron preparations are available in many different forms and may be sold over the counter.

Although most people get plenty of iron in their normal

diet, loss of blood may result in iron deficiency. This is particularly the case with women who lose iron during menstruation.

When extra iron is added to the diet for long periods of time, some of it may be deposited in the tissues of the body. Therefore doctors nowadays are careful to watch the use of iron by the patient, allowing intervals so as to permit the body to clear itself of excess.

VITAMINS

Vitamins, which are fully discussed in a chapter in this book, are widely used as home remedies to prevent vitamin deficiencies and also to maintain adequate amounts of vitamins in the body.

Scientific research has shown that vitamins are essential to maintain normal body chemistry. Most people who live on complete and well-balanced diets, including the seven basic foods, probably secure enough vitamins. However, the refining of foods and processes like heating, freezing, and other methods of packaging may injure to some extent the natural vitamin content. When baking soda is added to green vegetables to preserve their color while they are being cooked, some of the thiamine is destroyed. When vegetables are boiled, the water may dissolve out some of the vitamins and minerals.

Such major vitamin-deficiency diseases as beriberi, pellagra, and scurvy have been practically eliminated in the

United States. But many experts believe that minor deficiencies of these substances may unfavorably influence health.

A person on a restricted diet, either reducing, diabetic, or other, or a pregnant woman who loses her appetite, will get an insufficient amount of vitamins. Hence physicians are likely to prescribe vitamins for such people.

WEIGHT-CONTROL DRUGS

Among home products offered people who are reducing are drugs prescribed by the doctor which can interfere with appetite, sometimes thyroid materials when the thyroid supply is deficient, and occasionally products that add bulk in the intestines (of which, among others, are psyllium seeds and cellulose products, which draw water from the bowel and make up the bulk).

Many people nowadays buy fixed-formula diets of approximately nine hundred calories a day on which they may reduce without the danger of insufficient vitamins and minerals. Sugar may be lessened and the sense of sweetness satisfied by the use of preparations of saccharin or the cyclamates which are sold as Sucaryl®.

COLD AND COUGH REMEDIES

Among the most frequent of all conditions which people suffer are coughs and colds. The average American has from two to four colds a year with blocking of the nose, a mild fever, sometimes a cough. Scientists have shown that some eighty different viruses may be associated with the common cold. The preparation of vaccines against such a considerable number of viruses is almost impossible.

Most cold remedies, of which many are now freely available at the drugstore, are mixtures of pain relievers like aspirin or phenacetin, decongestant substances which stop the swelling in the nose, expectorant substances which loosen the secretions in the bronchial tubes, and antihistamines since many people are sensitive to various substances that are inhaled. Some of these mixtures also contain substances that act against cough. A cough is a reflex response to any irritation in the throat, the trachea, or the bronchial tubes. Such irritations are associated with infections, allergies, the presence of foreign substances like those that may be swallowed and stick in the throat. Coughs may also be associated with inflammations of the nerves in the throat or even with the growth of tumors.

Removal of the cause will stop the cough. Since removal of the cause may require some time, the discomfort of the cough meantime may be reduced by the usual cough remedies. However, any cough that persists for more than a few days should have analysis and treatment by a physician. Whereas most coughs are slight and likely to disappear in a few days, one must always remember that such conditions as tuberculosis, pneumonia, and tumors may produce persistent coughs.

Scientists talk about drugs that are "antitussive," which simply means that they are against cough. Many drugs have been developed that have proved capable of ameliorating conditions associated with coughing.

HAY-FEVER ALLEVIANTS
AND OTHER
ANTI-ALLERGY PREPARATIONS

Hay fever and asthma are frequent conditions affecting some millions of people. They represent sensitivities to various pollens that may be inhaled or to such foreign substances as animal hair or chemicals. Allergies may produce skin disturbances such as blisters or wheals (itching or burning spots) associated with the taking of foods to which the person may be sensitive. Generalized itching may be a response. Less serious is stuffiness in the nose and occasional swelling.

Most of the available home remedies are used to prevent the involvement of the sinuses, the sneezing, and the irritation and redness of the eyes that may come with allergies.

The chief constituents of the preparations used are decongestants and antihistamines. These preparations have been found helpful in what are called head colds, in vasomotor rhinitis, sinusitis, hay fever, and even in some cases when the ear reacts with congestion of the Eustachian tubes that pass from the throat to the ear.

LOCAL ANTISEPTICS

Among the most commonly used home remedies are mouthwashes and gargles. The old National Formulary contained a preparation called *liquor antisepticus,* an acid formula, and *liquor antisepticus alkalinus,* an alkaline formula. These preparations are now available in proprietary products which have the advantage of being carefully prepared, standardized, and distributed in acceptable packages.

More recently other antiseptic drugs have been discovered, some more efficient than those included in the older preparations. Thus the purchaser may have a choice, using the ones which have for him the most pleasant taste and the greatest acceptability.

Among the antiseptic substances recently developed are soaps with antiseptic ingredients, lotions which may contain alcohol that acts as an antiseptic, and all of the common antiseptics such as iodine, Mercurochrome®, hexylresorcinol, and many others. These efficient antiseptics have taken the place of the old boric-acid compounds which were only mildly antiseptic.

For certain special conditions sulphur combinations are available. Our food and drug laws also permit the inclusion of certain antibiotic drugs in antiseptic preparations that are applied to the skin for ringworm, burns, barber's itch, acne, impetigo, and other skin conditions.

The law does not permit purchases over the counter of antiseptic lotions to be put into the eye. There are good eyewashes that can help resolve congestion and redness, but any more potent drugs are reserved for prescription by the doctor.

TONICS

At the turn of the century many tonic preparations were sold containing iron, quinine, caffeine, and other drugs. Caffeine is a stimulant drug which is found in coffee and which is also included in various headache and similar preparations to counteract drowsiness and fatigue. Iron continues to be a basic constituent of tonics because many people have secondary anemias. Outside of such preparations the vitamins continue to be the most important tonic preparations. Among the vitamins, thiamine particularly has been shown by scientific study to have stimulating effects.

SEDATIVES AND TRANQUILIZERS

Among the great discoveries of recent years are the sedatives and the tranquilizers which differ from preparations of opium principally used for these purposes in a previous era. The newer drugs are seldom available without a doctor's prescription. However, some preparations of bromides are still available and also derivatives of scopolamine, the dosage being definitely limited to less than toxic doses. Some of these drugs act by producing forgetfulness which may well be an aid to sleep.

MOTION SICKNESS

For seasickness, airsickness, and car sickness, all of which are forms of motion sickness, new drugs have been introduced which in most countries can be bought without a prescription.

Some of these products have recently been said to be potentially harmful to pregnant women. They should not be taken by a pregnant woman unless specifically prescribed by the doctor.

A FEW WARNING NOTES

Among the classifications of drugs sold over the counter are, as already mentioned, the vitamins which come in a variety of mixtures designed for adults or for children and containing in some instances additional mineral salts, protein substances, and enzymes. These may be purchased without a physician's prescription, but you should ask the doctor if the particular formula chosen is suitable to your condition.

The cough and cold products include tablets, capsules, drops to be put in the nose, liquid preparations, materials to rub on the chest, formulas for coughs, lozenges, mists to be sprayed into the nose and throat, and gargles. For mild conditions these will usually be helpful. If a sore throat is not promptly relieved, study should be made by a doctor. If a cough persists more than a few days, a special examination is needed. Lozenges have a soothing quality and some of them are slightly anesthetic. In general they do not kill bacteria.

Chest rubs sometimes contain enough salicylates to have a slightly beneficial effect. They draw blood to the surface and produce a sense of warmth.

Nasal sprays are decongestant and antihistaminic. Overuse may be harmful.

The headache remedies are mostly based on aspirin with occasionally also phenacetin or modified acetanilid.

The claims that they go to any special portion of the nervous system and exert a specific effect are not well substantiated. In general, aspirin standardized according to the United States Pharmacopoeia has the same effects whether taken buffered, in capsules, in liquid, or in tablets, although some tablets tend to harden when kept long on the shelves and are not easily absorbed. Other pain-relieving substances are sometimes incorporated, but if in sufficient quantity to be effective may also be toxic.

Ointment, liniments, and other external medications may relieve burning or itching or inflammation, and occasionally are sufficiently antiseptic to destroy germs.

One should never attempt to treat a skin disturbance of the type of psoriasis without having an examination and prescription by a competent physician who understands diseases of the skin.

Preparations are also available for skins that are extra dry and for those that are extra oily, and these, in general, have value. Similarly many ointments are available for the treatment of burns. In mild burns most of these are helpful. Any severe burn that covers a considerable portion of the body should be cared for preferably in a hospital.

Great numbers of preparations are available for pimples and blackheads, but proper care of these conditions involves more than just smearing on an ointment.

Preparations for the care of the feet may be sold over the counter without a physician's prescription. Corn plasters depend principally on salicylic acid, which softens the tissue permitting the corn or callus to be removed. Foot powders will keep the skin dry and prevent spreading of infection and also relieve itching. Some contain specific substances that are antagonistic to ringworm. In severe and continued ringworm infestation potent products are now available, such as griseofulvin, which can be taken internally and prevent further growth and spread of ringworm.

A considerable number of preparations are listed under the heading "feminine hygiene." These include not only sanitary napkins and tampons but also douche powders and disinfectants which help to keep the organs clean and prevent infection. However, the rapid advance of medical science has made available specific drugs for the treatment of infectious organisms. These may be antiseptic or bacteriacidal. Certain infestations by flagellated organisms are now controllable by drugs like Metronidazole called Flagyl®. Most of the potent preparations can be prescribed only by a physician, but people should realize that such important products are available. The treatment for infestation with the organisms called trichomonas used to require repeated antiseptic douching and sometimes even surgical care, whereas nowadays most cases are relieved by use of the tablets of Metronidazole.

A great variety of suntan preparations are now available, all of which are safe when used as directed. These contain substances which inhibit the burning rays and tanning rays of the sun from acting on the skin. But some persons have extremely sensitive skins, and suntan lotion alone may not provide adequate protection against intensive sunlight.

Many deodorants may be purchased as creams, solutions, powders, sprays, and in other forms. Most of these depend for their effect on limiting the perspiration, on being astringent, and also on destroying certain germs on the skin. Cleanliness is essential to getting a completely satisfactory result with any deodorant.

Two
PAIN

More people go to see a doctor because of pain than for any other reason, and they are right to do so. Pain is an important warning signal. Few diseases develop without pain at some stage. Many involve so characteristic a pain as to make diagnosis certain. Whenever a pain is so severe, lasts so long, or is so unusual as to arouse alarm, a physician should be consulted. The famous Dr. Joseph Bloodgood once said that taking sodium bicarbonate to relieve the pain of an ulcer is like pouring water on the fire bell.

Yet there are times when it is perfectly safe and proper to use home remedies against pain, provided one knows the basic facts about pain and its function.

People vary greatly in their reaction to pain. Some suffer inordinately with pains that others disregard. Certain conditions of the mind may be accompanied by the illusion of physical pain. But it is a great mistake to conclude prematurely that someone's pain is imaginary. Every possible cause must be investigated before making the decision that the pain is related to hysteria or hypochondria.

One of the first problems is to make certain just where the pain is felt. Does it arise in the skin, or does it come from some of the organs inside the chest or abdomen? Pressure, warmth, or cold may cause pain. If the nerve endings are inflamed, pain is perceived at a lower threshold than normally.

Pain may be described as *pricking, burning, dull, intermittent,* or with many other words which define its character. A person may say that his pain is deep, by which he means under the skin. A burning pain, such as heartburn, may be related to irritation of the lower end of the esophagus.

Everybody has pains sometimes—the pain in the head that comes after eating ice cream or drinking cold water, a sudden pain in a muscle, the pain that is recognized as a rheumatic twinge. A "catch in the side" or "stitch" often attacks long-distance runners or others whose activity has put great demands on the oxygen of the body. This pain usually disappears when the runner gets what he calls his "second wind." These transitory pains are not cause for alarm and certainly should not lead to immediate ingestion of a pill. They usually go away, rarely return, and have little significance.

At the other end of the scale are the unusual, prolonged, or exceptionally severe pains that require attention from a physician. By appropriate examination he can tell whether the pain requires special attention or may be disregarded. Angina pectoris (literally "pain of the chest") is a heart pain that lasts two or three minutes and rarely more than ten or fifteen minutes. Identification is extremely important because special drugs are needed for relief, and the doctor's understanding and advice may prevent recurrence. The pain of a peptic ulcer may last an hour or more and may be relieved by taking some food or even a drink of water.

Only a doctor can recognize what are called referred pains. These are pains which originate at one point but which are felt at another point where they are carried by the nerves. A pain that persists over a long time, commonly called a chronic pain, may have most serious effects. A person with a continuous pain becomes irritated, easily tired, has difficulty in sleeping, loses appetite, and may, in fact, have what has been called either an anxiety state or a nervous breakdown.

TREATMENT OF PAIN

An analgesic is what doctors call a drug that relieves pain. Among the most widely used analgesics are aspirin and phenacetin, which are common constituents of most pain-relieving pills. Much stronger are such substances as codeine (derived from opium), the derivatives of barbituric acid (called barbiturates), and various other substances which act on the nervous system and which can be secured only with a doctor's prescription. Some of the substances called antihistamines or tranquilizers may also relieve pain, but these too in most instances require a doctor's prescription. Aspirin, whose scientific name is acetylsalicylic acid, is the most commonly used of all pain-relieving substances. It is also sold under a variety of trade names when it is modified by the addition of alkaline substances or by being put in capsules, or with a coating so that it will not act in the stomach but only when it reaches the intestine. Aspirin may be supplied in tablets, in capsules, or dissolved with other ingredients in a liquid.

Like other remedies, the dosages for children are smaller than for adults, but in proper dosage aspirin is safe even for infants. It is now available in various flavors and even in candied pills. This is a convenience, but it may also be a danger. The aspirin container should always be placed where children cannot reach it. Accidental poisonings from overdose of aspirin can be tragic.

Most common-cold pills contain aspirin and phenacetin. Caffeine may be added to counteract dullness or depression. In the United States it is not permissible to add codeine to such prescriptions. In Great Britain this is permitted, but the amount is limited to a definitely small dosage.

Three
HEADACHES

More than half the people who consult a doctor describe headache as one of their most distressing symptoms. Doctors in great industrial plants say that from 20–25 per cent of absences of employees are caused by headaches.

A committee established by the National Institute of Neurological Diseases and Blindness classified some two hundred possible causes of headache into a few main groups. Among these are nervous-tension headaches with contraction of neck muscles; migraine headaches of many different types; headaches associated with the eyes, ears, nose, sinuses, and throat; and headaches related to the brain itself. The cause of some headaches may be anywhere in the body rather than just in the head. Occasionally headaches are related to constipation, overeating, or indigestion. Since headaches have so many possible causes the best control is dependent on finding the cause and if possible removing it.

An occasional headache may be insignificant and unimportant. When headaches occur again and again, tending to localize in some single area of the head, relief of the pain is not enough. Such headaches demand special investigation by a physician.

Serious and persistent headaches may be caused by diseases of the kidney or the liver. Among other serious causes of headache are injuries to the head or diseases that affect the head.

The less serious headache such as that which comes with the ordinary cold, is probably due to congestion in the mucous membranes of the nose and sinuses. Such congestion may close the opening of the sinuses and prevent drainage. Possibly a partial vacuum created by the congestion may pull on the mucous membranes of the sinuses. This irritates the nerve endings and results in a dull pain over the eyebrows. If the frontal sinus, located in the forehead over the eyes, is involved, the ache is worse in the morning and lessens or disappears during the day as the sinuses drain into the nose. Nose drops or inhalations are used to shrink the swollen membranes and reduce the congestion of the sinuses, permitting air to enter. This will greatly lessen the pain and promote drainage.

Headaches from eyestrain are less common than popularly believed. Such headaches, which also usually occur at the forehead, may afflict children after being in school all day. If, however, a person has nearsighted, farsighted, astigmatic, or otherwise abnormal eyes not properly corrected by glasses or contact lenses, the continued strain associated with seeing may result in headache. Suitable eyeglasses to correct the defect remove strain and headache.

Toxic headaches result from a great variety of substances such as alcohol, gases, drugs, tobacco, or other substances that can affect the circulation of blood in the brain. A common example is the headache one gets after missing an accustomed cup of coffee in the morning.

Migraine is a special form of headache which fortunately is not as common as vascular and nervous headaches. It comes on suddenly as intense pain usually on one side of the head. Some people can feel it coming on and by lying down and taking aspirin prevent the attack or reduce its intensity. Severe and repeated migraine requires a physician's care, since the remedies for it have to be taken under professional supervision.

Still other headaches are called *functional*, because a definite cause cannot be found for them. Such headaches may be associated with high or low blood pressure, anemia, excessive emotional strain, fatigue, premenstrual tension, or various forms of allergy.

Psychologists recognize a form of headache called *psychogenic*, which is associated with excessive emotion. The specialist in psychosomatic medicine suggests that if a person has unconsciously hated someone for a long time, he may respond with a headache every time he sees that person. While one should hardly jump to the conclusion that secret love, hate, anger, rage, or laughter causes every headache, still, in the absence of any other determinable cause, a psychogenic cause may be suspected.

The *nervous tension* or *emotional* headaches are most common and are produced when the muscles in the back of the head and neck become tense from tension or emotion. This is felt in the head as a dull aching pain. These headaches are about four times as frequent in women as in men. Headache specialists have reported that more than two thirds of all headaches are of this kind.

TREATMENT

Conceivably a dull throb in the head at the end of a hard day's work may result from a combination of fatigue, hunger, and strain. A little food will relieve the hunger. Loosening the clothing and relaxing the muscles may help the strain, and rest will overcome the fatigue. The application of a cold compress over the eyes and forehead helps. After a little rest, a brisk walk and change of scene or an alternating warm and cold shower may stimulate the circulation and help the headache.

If the cause of the headache is mainly congestion of blood and fluid in the head, a hot foot bath may draw blood from this congested area and make the headache disappear.

Even migraine may respond to treatment rather easily. According to a distinguished professor of medicine at Oxford University, Dr. George Pickering, some cases require no treatment beyond an explanation to the patient and reassurance that the attacks will not result in permanent harm. Some people are quick to recognize for themselves the kind of incidents that bring on an attack and try to avoid them.

For less easily treated, but not severe migraines, the same drugs which the patient takes for himself for milder forms of headaches are applicable. In severe migraine cases physicians usually have to use drugs derived from ergot in addition to the usual headache remedies.

Since most headaches are associated with tension and sometimes with mental depression, many commonly used drugs may be helpful. Caffeine is a drug which helps to constrict the blood vessels and thus reduce flow of blood in the brain. It may be combined in the treatment of nervous-tension headaches with pain-relieving drugs such as aspirin and phenacetin. The nervous-tension component is also helped by small doses of mild tranquilizers which can be obtained in combination with aspirin and other drugs without a prescription. Because of possible effects not directly related to the headaches, larger doses of tranquilizers should be taken only when prescribed by the doctor.

But the main weapon in stopping painful headache is aspirin. It may be used also in various combination products such as with phenacetin, caffeine or tranquilizers, effervescent formulas, or tablets containing alkalis. The usual adult dose is five or ten grains, that is, one or two tablets. Since more than two tablets usually do not give greater headache relief than the two-tablet dose, more than two are not needed.

For small children the dose must be adjusted, following closely the directions given on the label of the bottle. Children's size tablets are usually $1\frac{1}{4}$ grains, that is, one quarter the size of the adult tablet. Mothers should be careful not to give their children larger doses of such products than are advised on the label.

Infants are much more susceptible to aspirin than larger children. Under three years old a child can only be treated safely with aspirin by a physician. The first symptom of overdosage with aspirin in an infant is excessive restlessness and rapid forced breathing. Any such symptoms, where overdosage is suspected, require immediate attention by a physician even if the infant otherwise does not seem to be seriously sick.

I repeat here: the warning on the aspirin bottle, "Keep this and all medicines out of the reach of children," should be carefully heeded. A large number of toddling infants and small children are poisoned each year by medicine or household products left carelessly within their reach.

Another important caution calls for discontinuing self-medication if the condition lasts more than ten days without relief. Also pointed out on many labels is the fact that headache from severe sore throat with fever requires a physician's expert care, as does the pain of severe rheumatism and arthritis.

Four
BACKACHE

Evolutionists believe that man was once an animal on four legs who forced himself to stand on two in order to be able to use his arms and hands. Even today, after long ages, we may not be completely adjusted to the upright posture.

Women, especially, are prone to backache. The spines of man and woman are curved differently, because the lower end of the spine in woman is more horizontal than in man. Anything that increases this angle produces strain on the ligaments, and with strain comes pain. During pregnancy the ligaments loosen. After the baby is born, they usually become tight again but sometimes they do not. This too may cause pain.

There are many more sources of backache. When one leg is shorter than the other, which is not uncommon, the pelvis tilts, causing strain and pain. People who assume slouchy positions in sitting and standing finally force the back into a bad position for carrying stress. Fallen arches

44

may cause pain in the lower part of the back. Shoes that do not permit proper balance, such as extra high heels, may result in backache. Any job that makes the worker frequently assume positions that are unnatural or which throws excessive loads on different parts of the body for long periods will irritate the joints of the knee, the hip, and the spine. People who stand or kneel at work are subject to pains in the back.

Apart from these simple mechanical difficulties, the spine may be subject to disease. As with other parts of the body, infections, tumors, softening of the bones, and inflammations of the joint tissues may result in pain. Between the bones of the back are little cartilages which act as cushions. These are called disks. If a disk gets out of place, it gets pinched and pain results. Since the nerves of the body come out in the spaces between the bones, they get pinched and pain follows. Sometimes extension of the spine will relieve this pain, but sometimes surgery may be necessary.

Pain in the back may be referred from the prostate gland, an ulcer of the stomach, hemorrhoids, infections or inflammations of the organs of women associated with childbirth. Contrary to some people's belief, the kidneys are not a primary cause of pain in the back.

When a person has persistent pain in the back, a physician should be consulted who will provide for X-ray study. But often a backache will respond to such simple measures as the use of a board to stiffen the mattress, or the application of heat by an electric pad or hot-water bottle.

The drugs people try for backache are the same as those used for headache: the simple pain relievers like aspirin in various forms and mixtures of aspirin with phenacetin and caffeine.

Some people find relief from backache by the application of cold, using an icebag. After the third or fourth day, heat may be substituted for the cold to improve the circulation and to relax the muscle spasm which develops to counteract the pain.

Recently developed drugs include special antispasmodic drugs specifically designed to relieve muscle spasm and which the physician will prescribe if he feels that they are needed. Occasionally supporting garments are used which take the pull and strain off the joints in the spine.

Sometimes people under stress who have backache obtain temporary relief from tranquilizing and anxiety-relieving drugs. However, any backache that persists should lead to proper investigation and proper treatment.

Five
SLEEPLESSNESS AND
SLEEPING PILLS

Everybody has his own ideas about sleep, and no wonder. By the time he is thirty years old, the average person has had more than twelve solid years of experience with slumber.

Up to age thirty most people have little trouble with sleep. Perhaps before an exam in school or college, or the night before a proposal, or before playing in a big game, a younger person may toss about a bit. But most often he merely drops into bed, fits himself into his usual sleeping position, and next thing he knows the sunlight is streaming in and the birds chirping.

By age thirty most people have developed a technique or routine of sleep. Each has a favorite hour of retirement, a favorite bed, a favorite posture, and a favorite formula. A collection of such habits makes up the routine of falling asleep. During rest—particularly the rest that comes with sleep—the fatigue of the body disappears and recuperation begins. A tired mind gathers new force.

The memory improves. Annoyances and problems which loomed large on going to bed are seen in better perspective.

Investigators have tried to find out how long a person can go without sleep. Several people have reached more than 115 hours, nearly five days. The limit, whatever it may be for an individual, is absolute. Animals kept awake for from five to eight days have died of exhaustion. Probably a week is the outside limit for human beings.

Stories are told of many noted people who slept but little. Napoleon, Edison, Darwin, and others reputedly averaged four to six hours a night. Since age eighteen I have myself averaged only six hours a night. Some people do well with little sleep; others require eight to ten hours in each twenty-four. Infants sleep sixteen to eighteen hours, the period gradually diminishing. The schoolboy or schoolgirl may take twelve hours. The high school and college student may need ten. The worker with a physically demanding job may need ten, while the high-pressure, dynamic executive may manage on six to eight.

Does rest without sleep aid in overcoming fatigue and exhaustion? Definitely. An hour in the middle of the day in a recumbent position is a marvelous restorative of flagging energy. Three hours of quiet, undisturbed sleep may be more refreshing than eight hours of tossing around. Three or four hours at home in one's accustomed bed may produce more recuperation than ten hours on a moving train. A few hours of normal sleep may do much more for health than many hours of unconsciousness induced by drugs.

Habit and the mental state are the most important elements in sleep production. The man who has lived a regular life and who invariably shuts the door and tries the lock, winds the clock, opens the window, pulls down the shade, and climbs into bed from a certain side finds himself making the motions unnecessarily if some of the appurtenances are absent. If the clock has been sent for repairs, he is likely to reach for it just the same. So accustomed does he become to certain sounds that their absence interferes with sleep. Silence becomes obtrusive. The visitor to the city is kept awake by the elevated railway, the street cars, or the apartment elevator. But the city apartment dweller who never notices these sounds paces the floor distractedly during his first few nights in the country, cursing the frogs and katydids.

Many scientific studies have been made of the intensity of sleep. All of the evidence seems to indicate that you sleep most soundly during the first few hours and that the depth of sleep diminishes toward morning. In the language of the psychiatrists, the threshold for stimuli is lowered. Much is made, therefore, of controlling noises of all sorts during sleeping hours. Even during sleep the mind seems to be attuned, like a radio, to certain wave lengths. The mother whose rest is unaffected by the roar of a passing train is awakened by the whimper of her child.

In general the less noise, the better sleep. Unusual

noises are the worst disturbers. Loose boards, loose shutters and windows, creaking springs, shaky fixtures, leaky faucets may need to be checked. But light is also a stimulus. Indeed some people can sleep in the daytime only when all light is sealed out by opaque shades and hangings. Everything in the room that might reflect light—mirrors, pictures, polished brass of a bed—may have to be studied.

We may also be disturbed through our senses of smelling, temperature, skin perception, equilibrium, or position in space. For hygienic sleeping the temperature of the room should range from sixty to seventy degrees F., although one can easily accustom oneself to sleeping at lower temperatures. It is particularly difficult to sleep when the body is kept too warm and evaporation from its surface prevented by too much or too thick a covering. Babies have to be kept warmer than adults. The air should be fresh and in motion, but drafts should be avoided. A sudden draft of cold air will awaken a sleeper.

It is certainly true that one sleeps best in the bed to which one is accustomed, but there is an important qualification. How old is the bed? Springs sag; mattresses bunch in spots; beds loosen, wobble, and creak with age; pillows lose resilience. When springs sag so badly that one sleeps as if in a hammock, it is time to change; the human body has not been developing toward that conformation. Since one is likely to move about when receiving a stimulus to the skin or to the muscles during sleep, such stimuli must be avoided. The mattress should, therefore, be soft enough to give in response to the movement of the body and hard enough to support the body and not permit it to move too much. The bed clothing should be light in weight and free of wrinkles. It should not be drawn so tight as to hinder motion, since sleep experiments have shown that a sleeper may change positions from thirty to one hundred times in eight hours without awakening.

With the temperature and humidity salubrious, with the bed comfortable, with noise and light and odors and tactile perceptions fully controlled, the sleeper lies down at his accustomed hour and falls asleep. That is to say, he falls asleep if everything is satisfactory to him mentally. As Hamlet says, "Ay, there's the rub!"

A mind sufficiently under control can discount strange surroundings, noises, odors, sleeping garments, and many other physical stimuli. It must also be sufficiently under control to discard memories, worries, anger, love, and particularly fear. The habit of discarding mental stimuli on going to bed must either be established when young or learned by much discipline of the mind later. In the presence of serious fear—fear of death of one's loved ones, fear of discovery of falsehood, crime, or deceit, fear of loss of job, or of money, or of failure of courage in battle or in sport, sleep stays away. It stays away at the time when it is needed most. Then one conjures it back—or tries to inveigle it—by formulas. One reads dull books, one counts sheep, one breathes rhythmically—the methods for diverting attention are legion.

Insomnia has been described as inability to sleep due to real or imaginary causes. Anxieties of any kind can cause the mind to dwell upon them so constantly as to make sleep difficult, and automatically create a new anxiety—the anxiety as to whether sleep will or will not come. Another form of insomnia is waking up too soon, accompanied by inability to fall asleep again.

The person who wakes up in time to begin the day's activities has generally had enough sleep. However, people who persistently wake up too early for breakfast, the morning paper, and going to work, and at the same time feel tired and depressed, should consult a physician.

People who need only six hours of sleep should avoid going to bed before midnight. A revised old proverb says, "Early to bed, early to rise and you meet no prominent people." If you need six hours of sleep and you go to bed at ten, you will find few people to talk to at four o'clock in the morning.

WHAT ABOUT DRUGS?

Drugs are a crutch which should only be used as a last resort. Most of the drugs that are really effective must be prescribed by a doctor. Before asking your doctor for a prescription, try the sedative effect of a hot bath, a hot drink, an electric blanket, or a hot-water bottle, and check to make sure you are avoiding such physical stimuli as indigestible food, or coffee, tea, and caffeine-containing soft drinks near bedtime.

The doctors have a wide variety of drugs for prescription to the person who needs them to establish proper sleep habits. Some are powerful enough to be dangerous, and the laws in many countries make it difficult for doctors to prescribe them and druggists to dispense them.

But even drugs that are sedative in small doses become hypnotics when taken in large doses. The leading class of drugs for these purposes is the barbiturates. There are many kinds of barbiturates—some that act slowly for a long time and others that act quickly for a short time. People should also be aware of the tranquilizing drugs which may reduce tension and anxiety and thus aid sleep.

One of the difficulties with all these drugs is that they may induce dependence to such an extent that you become a habitual user and cannot get to sleep without them. As with cathartics and laxatives, the aim should be by proper use of the drugs to restore normal habits free of dependence on drugs.

If the doctor finds that failure to sleep is due to pain, he can prescribe drugs that will relieve the pain. If coughing interferes with sleep, treatment of the cough is more satisfactory than taking a sleeping pill.

Several non-barbiturate drugs are now available that can be bought under trade names without a doctor's prescription. However, the doctor's advice should be sought even before trying any of these.

GADGETRY OF SLEEP

A New York City shop is devoted entirely to gadgets to aid people who find sleeping difficult. One of the simplest is two plugs of cotton that fit into the ears. For people who are disturbed by light, sleep shades and sleep masks are available, the latter in a variety of designs including quilted satin with colored embroideries, and even monograms.

For people who like to fall asleep listening to soft music, radios with clock mechanisms automatically shut off after a certain length of time. Special records and tapes for insomniacs offer soothing sounds, soothing music, and monotonous suggestions. People who become addicted to falling asleep by this technique sometimes discover that they cannot attend a concert without dropping off.

More recently massage and heat mattress pads have been developed which can vibrate one into restfulness. Not long ago I dropped a quarter in a device in a hotel with the idea that I would test the vibrating mattress. Nothing happened. Some hours later I suddenly wakened with the feeling that an earthquake was occurring. The current which had been off when I went to bed had belatedly gone into action.

SNORING

When you consider that modern noise-measuring machines have clocked snores at forty decibels—the equivalent of a noisy office or a roaring motor car—you can understand why snoring creates such a disturbance. Is snoring necessary? Is there any sure cure for it?

Well, there are different kinds of snoring, and they have different causes. No single "cure" fits all of them. But the belief of many snorers that they just can't help it is unwarranted. If anyone really wants to stop snoring, he should first find out why he snores, and then try to remove the cause.

A familiar theory of snoring is that the soft palate relaxes, particularly when a person is lying on his back, and partially obstructs the nasal passage, so that air passing through causes a noisy vibration. But that explanation is inadequate. Physiologists point out that the soft palate may vibrate when a sleeper inhales, but that when he exhales it would be likely to close the nasal passage, preventing air from passing through. And yet people snore when exhaling, too. The truth is that the soft palate is only one of the possible noisemakers. Others are: relaxation of the muscles governing the vocal cords, presence of mucus in the nasal passages, the falling backward of the tongue, and other abnormal conditions.

Abnormal conditions are, of course, cases for a physician; and chronic snorers should have a checkup. A nose-and-throat specialist tells me that a man recently came to him shamefaced and said his wife insisted that he be examined because of his snoring. "She's a musician," he explained, "and she wouldn't mind so much except that I keep getting off pitch." The physician found that the wall between the man's nostrils was curved out of line. When this condition was corrected by surgery, the man no longer snored, either flat, sharp, or on pitch. That is one of several abnormal possibilities. In children, removal of adenoids is often recommended.

Most ordinary snoring is caused either by muscular relaxation or by mucus in the nasal passages, or both. Many snorers would be insulted if told the truth—that they can stop snoring by making sure that their noses and throats are clean before going to bed. Mucus irritation, of course, can come from many causes: colds, catarrhal conditions, sinus infections. Recently it has been found that allergies to some foods may set up mucus irritations and cause snoring.

I knew a man who insisted that getting bald made him a snorer. He argued that when he lost his hair his head was no longer protected from the night air: that he caught cold, got stuffed up—and snored. The colds probably did have a lot to do with his snoring, though I suspect the bald head was innocent.

Relaxation, however, probably remains the chief contributory cause of snoring. Scientists who have studied snoring report:

That babies, unable to control their muscles, snore frequently.

That adolescents and younger adults, having firm muscles, seldom snore.

That snoring increases from the age of thirty on, because of letdown in muscular control.

The relaxation that seems most definitely to start the snoring comes when sleeping on the back. Then the soft palate or vocal cords are most likely to fall into an obstructive position, the jaw may fall, causing mouth breathing—and the nocturnal rumpus starts.

Many devices have been rigged up through the years to try to prevent snoring. Most of them are based on the sound theory that most snoring would be eliminated if people would keep off their backs and breathe through their noses. One of the earliest was a spool tied around the waist on a string, and placed in the middle of the back. This certainly would keep a man off his back—or a woman, for that matter, because women do snore too. Other devices that have been tried include baseballs sewed into little pockets in the back of sleeping garments, pillows propped up in such a way as to keep the sleeper from turning over.

Recent investigators have learned a number of interesting things about sleepers and snorers. Old people sleep less deeply than do young ones. Sleep apparently becomes deepest during the first hour and progressively less deep from that time on. Non-snorers sleep better than snorers. Snorers are likely to sleep with the mouth open, while those who do not snore sleep with the mouth closed and breathe through the nose. Scientists do not relate snoring to sleeping with the mouth open, but they do relate it to breathing through the mouth as a habit. They do not feel that snoring is a measure of depth of sleep because some of the people who snored and who slept lightly during the first stages of sleep slept more deeply after they stopped snoring.

Six
ANTI-INFECTIVE DRUGS

A wide variety of antiseptics is available in drugstores to combat infection in the nose and throat and on the skin.

Cleanliness, particularly the use of soap and water with a brush or a washcloth, is an excellent antiseptic procedure for the skin. However, this will not destroy many dangerous germs or parasites. Hence the development of antiseptic solutions.

Iodine is one of the most efficient substances for killing germs. Ordinary tincture of iodine has, therefore, been widely used. When the preparation contains more than 2 per cent iodine, it may be irritating. Instead of being dissolved in alcohol, as it is in a tincture, iodine may be dissolved in water, making it less irritating.

Various preparations of mercury used as antiseptics are also easily available. Among them are Mercurochrome®, Metaphen®, and Merthiolate®. These are not irritating. They do possess some antiseptic action, although it has been attributed by some experts to the alcohol in which the drug substance is dissolved.

Various forms of silver have been used, such as silver nitrate and the preparation called argyrol. However, silver has fallen into some disrepute among doctors as an antiseptic. One of the dangers of using silver is a permanent discoloration of the skin, a condition called argyria.

Among the most commonly used antiseptics are the alcohols, not only ethyl alcohol but also isopropyl alcohol. These destroy ordinary germs. A 50 per cent alcohol solution is just about as effective as pure alcohol. Such substances are often used for body rubs during long illnesses.

Another popular antiseptic is hydrogen peroxide, which performs a cleansing action by dissolving dead tissue. Drugs which develop oxygen, such as potassium permanganate and sodium perborate, have been effectively used against certain afflictions, permanganate against ringworm and sodium perborate for mouth cleansing, particularly against Vincent's organisms, which cause the condition called trench mouth.

A great variety of soaps have mild antiseptic action as well as non-irritating detergent action.

Still another group of antiseptics are the ammonia compounds, most of which are available for purchase. Among those sold under trade names are Zephiran®, Phemerol®, Ceepryn®, and Triburon®. A form of ammonia known as methyl benzethonium, commonly called

Diaparene®, is used to prevent skin irritation from the urine of babies who wear diapers.

Doctors are wary of strong antiseptic substances like carbolic acid or phenol, which are dangerous when spilled on the skin in pure form and may easily be irritating even when diluted. Moreover, many cases of accidental poisoning from phenol have occurred. The cresols have also been used. These are derived from phenol.

Among recent antiseptics is hexachlorophene, which has become an ingredient of many mouthwashes and antiseptic solutions, and even of soaps. Among the products based on hexachlorophene are Gamophen®, pH iso-Hex®, and many well-known soaps.

The value of boric acid as an antiseptic is limited. Its antiseptic properties are weak, and in addition it may be dangerous. Deaths of infants have occurred from taking boric acid accidentally, and even from absorption through the skin.

MOUTHWASHES AND GARGLES

For years doctors have argued the value of mouthwashes and gargles. Many have insisted that a mouthwash does nothing but wash out loose material and replace temporarily the odor that is there with its own odor. However, extensive testing of many mouthwashes has now shown their ability actually to destroy germs, and many people have come to depend on the use of mouthwashes to control bad breath. For some time attempts were made to use chlorophyll tablets, but thus far real proof that these can remove odor from the breath is not available.

The commonest causes of bad breath are infection in the mouth, nose, sinuses, throat, air passages, or lungs, or the presence of debris from food between the teeth. Alcoholic liquors, garlic, and onions are common causes.

Decayed teeth and infection of the gums also are associated with bad breath. These require a visit to the dentist. Modern dental cleansing involves removal of tartar from the teeth by scaling, which is also sometimes sufficient to control bad breath. Regular washing of the teeth with an acceptable toothpaste and brush, particularly after eating, is useful. However, just as mouthwashes cleanse only temporarily, because new food and inhalation of air come very promptly after the teeth have been washed, there is some doubt that the effects of some toothpastes linger longer than those of others.

The mouthwashes most widely used in the United States include, among others, Listerine®, Micrin®, Borolyptol®, Cepryl®, Steri/Sol®, Lavoris®, Isodine®, Green Mint®, and Colgate's Oral Antiseptic®.

Seven
THE COMMON COLD

The average child has at least four colds a year, the average adult at least two, but individuals vary widely. Why some people are much more susceptible than others is not yet certain. Apparently the fact is related to that poorly defined constitutional condition called resistance. Research has shown that as many as eighty different viruses may be associated with the common cold, along with a variety of secondary germ invaders.

Colds are highly contagious, passing rapidly from one person to another in a family, a factory, a classroom, or just about any place where people assemble. The incidence of colds is lowest in summer, rises in the fall, reaches a peak in midwinter, and declines with the coming of spring. A lesser peak is reached in the fall when schools open and children assemble in classrooms.

Much attention has been given to whether air drafts, or getting hot and then being exposed to cold, may bring on a common cold. Many serious investigations have been made in an attempt to prove the effects of such factors, but thus far even the simplest questions remain without answer.

A cold usually begins suddenly with a sense of soreness and dryness in the nose or in the back of the throat. Within a few hours the nasal passages feel congested, sneezing develops, and a colorless, watery discharge comes from the nose. After about forty-eight hours the cold reaches its peak. Then comes excessive watering of the eyes, huskiness of the voice, and difficulty in breathing. This is due to congestion. With the coming of secondary germs, the nasal discharge becomes thick and sticky. If the secretions drop into the throat, a cough develops. These coughs do not bring up much discharge unless the person has some chronic inflammation of the bronchial tubes. With the invasion of the viruses and the germs some fever may develop, in children, particularly, reaching occasionally as high as 102 or 103 degrees. The congestion of the nose is often accompanied by a headache. As with most minor infections, there may be some drowsiness and feeling of illness, vague pains in the back and in the limbs.

An uncomplicated cold generally lasts from one to two weeks. Colds which persist or recur repeatedly or in which there is a steady, prolonged fever or chills may indicate complications. If a cold persists longer than two weeks, a physician should certainly be consulted.

Attempts have been made to develop a vaccination against colds. These have been without success, although some vaccines are available against certain types of influenza.

The prevention of colds is not specific. The measures usually used to ward off infection and reduce the frequency of colds are those said to produce increased resistance. A well-balanced diet, sufficient rest, and proper clothing to keep the body warm outdoors or cool indoors are said to help raise resistance. Even though proof is not available about changes in temperature, undue exposure to sharp changes in temperature should be avoided. Some evidence exists that the mucous membranes are affected by such changes, reducing their resistance to infection. If rooms are properly ventilated, with sufficient humidity in the air, the mucous membranes are aided in maintaining a healthy condition. American homes are usually overheated. If humidifiers are not used, moisture may be improved by keeping a pan of water on a radiator or stove.

One ought to keep away from people who have bad colds, but under modern conditions of civilization in our cities such avoidance of contact is just about impossible. If a husband or wife develops a severe cold, they might temporarily sleep in separate rooms, but the contact will usually have been made before the cold developed fully. Perhaps husbands and wives should simply reconcile themselves to the fact that when one has a cold, the other will probably get it. Nevertheless, the basic hygienic measures like washing the hands before eating and using a handkerchief to cover a sneeze can be helpful in reducing spread of colds within a family.

TREATMENT

If a cold is severe, it is a good idea to stay home for a brief period, preferably in bed. This not only permits the body maximal recovery but helps prevent spreading the cold to one's fellow workers. Other hygienic measures include plenty of liquids (hot or cold), a light diet, and keeping warm.

Innumerable remedies are available in drugstores for self-treatment of colds. Aspirin, the universal pain reliever, may be taken in one of numerous forms. It does not cure colds by destroying the viruses or the germs, but it does help relieve the indefinite pains and perhaps helps to keep the fever down. The United States Pharmacopoeia has established standards for aspirin, whether in tablets, capsules, or other forms. Not much difference, if any, exists among them. Some preparations are promoted with the claim that they produce less irritation of the stomach, but this has not been proved. Aspirin does not increase the acidity within the stomach; therefore combinations of aspirin with bicarbonate of soda and similar alkaline substances with the idea that this will result in less irritation of the stomach seem to be unnecessary. If a person has some irritation after taking aspirin, the cause lies elsewhere than in the aspirin. If combinations of other drugs with aspirin seem to lessen this irritation, the reason is probably that these drugs empty the stomach more rapidly. Some evidence exists that an aspirin tablet—or indeed a tablet of any kind—may get caught in the folds of the stomach or the intestine and produce irritation. Under such circumstances the condition is promptly discovered because of the irritation. However, some physicians are convinced that people who have irritation will probably do better if they can take the aspirin or other salicylates in a liquid mixture or in an effervescent aspirin tablet, or by crushing the aspirin tablet to a powder and mixing with orange juice, tomato juice, or some other drink.

In a recent discussion of the treatment of the common cold, Dr. Perrin H. Long has recommended that the person who has even a little fever when suffering from a cold should go to bed for a day or two—but few people do.

If the throat is sore, gargling may give a little relief. Great numbers of gargles are now available, such as Listerine®, Cepacol®, and Micrin®, which are designed to reduce the irritation in the throat associated with a cold. The pharmacist may help in selecting one. Old-time family remedies included gargling salt water, or even hot milk and other warm drinks.

Many of the preparations offered for a cold contain antihistaminic drugs. The chief value of these is that they dry the secretions. A directory of such preparations includes several hundred. Most contain chlorpheniramine maleate or phenyl propanolamine hydrochloride, among the most widely known being Coriforte®, Ornade®, and Sinutab®. These products are not available in some states without a doctor's prescription. The physician may recommend the dosage and duration of treatment.

Also important in relieving the symptoms of a cold are inhaling preparations and sprays which relieve congestion.

Colds have been catalogued as head colds, spring colds, summer colds and many others. Occasionally symptoms resembling those of a cold are associated with sensitization to the inhalation of various foreign protein substances which produce a histamine reaction. The condition may be called vasomotor rhinitis or "hay fever." This is associated with a running nose, congestion, tears, and similar reactions. Most of the common cold remedies include an antihistamine which would be helpful in such cases.

The doctor is constantly concerned about whether or not to prescribe for a cold a drug like a sulfonamide, penicillin, or other antibiotic. Most medical opinion now holds that these drugs should not be given routinely but only when there is evidence of secondary infection by germs and possible extension of these germs to the bronchial tubes, the sinuses, or the ears.

In the Armed Forces and in industrial plants the common treatment of a cold is a capsule or tablet containing what is called APC—a mixture of aspirin, phenacetin, and caffeine. Such mixtures are also available in a variety of forms in any drugstore. Many industrial physicians recommend that the person with a cold begin for the first few days with these drugs; then when the secretions in the nose get thick, any of the drops that contain 1 per cent ephedrine, used either in an atomizer or as nose drops, will help to relieve the congestion. Among those most frequently used are Neosynephrine®, Paredrine Hydrobromide®, and Tyzine®. When giving nose drops to a child, have the child tilt the head back; hold the head firmly. A good technique is to allow the hand that holds the dropper to rest on the head of the child. The number of drops recommended on the package can then be given successfully.

People often ask whether a child who has frequent colds should have tonsils and adenoids removed. That question can be answered only by a physician after examination to determine whether the infection and swelling are sufficient to demand removal of these tissues. When the tonsils and adenoids are so inflamed as to interfere with breathing, self-treatment is likely to be ineffective.

Attempts have been made to show that vitamins are related to frequency of catching cold and that, therefore, people who have colds ought to take mixed vitamins. Scientific evidence proves that the lack of any specific vitamin may predispose the person to infection through lowering the resistance. However, there is no scientific evidence that extra vitamins administered to a person free of deficiency disease will protect against respiratory infection. In other words, if you and your family are getting enough vitamins already, extra ones won't help you.

A wide variety of cough and cold products are now sold in American drugstores—far too many to be listed. Most of them are designed to lessen the coughing and to relieve other symptoms as much as possible. None can be considered a cure for a cough. Most consist of combinations of drugs, principally aspirin, occasionally an antihistamine or anti-allergy drug, sometimes a mild anesthetic preparation, sometimes simply syrup or other thick fluid which will coat the irritated membranes. A few contain sedatives. Anyone who buys a cough remedy should be sure to read the label and understand what he is taking.

Eight
CONSTIPATION

When food is taken into the mouth, digestion of starch begins with the saliva; other digestive fluids act in the stomach; the food is moved on into the small intestine for further digestive actions; then the residue moves on into the cecum and the large intestines, finally being passed from the body by way of the sigmoid and the rectum. In a normal person the activity becomes habitual, so that once or twice each day the bowel is emptied. Some people skip one or several days and are not in the slightest disturbed unless they begin to worry and become over-conscious of the condition. Then they begin to study their symptoms, carefully observe the results of every action of the bowel, strain and strive unnecessarily to force activity, and sooner or later develop the habit of taking too much roughage, too many pills, and too much trouble altogether. One doctor has suggested that the term constipation be abandoned altogether and that the phrase "colon-conscious" be substituted for it.

In general physicians are inclined to label a condition constipation when there is passage of unduly hard and dry material. The consistency of the material is more important than the frequency of the action. The motions of the intestinal tract vary with different people. The stomach empties in from two to seven hours. The time required for digestion in the small intestine is less—usually two to four hours. Then the residue enters the cecum, the first portion of the large bowel, in a liquid state. In the large bowel fluid is removed so that the material becomes more solid as it moves forward. When the mass reaches the sigmoid and rectum a nervous stimulus inclining toward emptying reaches the tissues. From one to three days is the usual time for passage through the large bowel, but even four or five days may be required.

When the material from the bowel is watery and unformed the condition is called diarrhea. When there is an excessive amount of gas, the diet and the speed of movement of the material through the colon may be responsible.

Usually constipation can be overcome by including adequate amounts of laxative foods in the diet. Oatmeal for breakfast or the use of whole wheat; spinach, prunes, figs, vegetables and fruits, honey and syrup are helpful. In the more severe cases the use of various oils, enemas, laxatives, or yeast may be tried.

Sir Arthur F. Hurst, one of the leading British authorities on gastrointestinal diseases, divides most cases of constipation into two varieties. In the first the colon or large bowel is at fault, and in the second the condition is related to the lower portion of the bowel, including the sigmoid and rectum.

Delay in passage of material through the colon may be due to deficient motor activity or to the fact that the nature of the material to be moved requires excessive force. When the food contains too little indigestible residue and when insufficient quantity of material is formed on an adequate diet, it is difficult for the muscles and nervous system of the bowel to act efficiently.

In very old people and in those who are undernourished, the muscle of the intestinal wall fails to develop or to keep its normal physical condition. Investigations show also that a lack of some of the vitamins of the B complex may be related to undernourishment and to failure of the bowel to act properly.

When the material passing through the bowel is abnormally dry, due either to insufficient consumption of water or to overproduction of sweat because of hot weather, there may be constipation because of the failure of the muscles of the bowel to have proper material on which to exercise their activity.

In the second type of constipation the proper nerve-muscle relationships fail to occur in the lower portion of the bowel. The baby can be trained so that the simple act of exposure and placing it on the pot will cause it to evacuate.

Older people develop a series of habits that are much more complicated. There is the matter of getting up, tak-

73

ing a bath, dressing, having breakfast and, finally, the question of access to the toilet, the provision of suitable reading matter, and a pipe or a cigarette. Already it is known that interference with any one of the factors of this involved series may disturb the whole mechanism.

The complication of nerve and muscle reaction is called a conditioned reflex. In most cases this kind of constipation or dyschesia results from neglect in responding to the call because of laziness, false modesty, bad discipline, or any one of a number of similar factors. Eventually failure to respond to the call to empty the bowel will result in loss of sensation. Unfortunately, however, by this time the person concerned has begun to fix his mind on his difficulties and is likely to begin indulging in laxatives, enemas, colon washings, or similar procedures which create new habits and result ultimately in a complete loss of the possibility of normal emptying of the bowel.

There are rare instances in which dyschesia may result from weakness of muscles, the fear of pain because of some disease in the area concerned, or even difficulties involving the nervous system, but these are rare compared with the vast majority of cases which result from bad habits.

In many instances people who are constipated have developed a fixation on the time, the amount, the shape, the color, or other factors associated with evacuation of the bowel. One of the first steps in overcoming constipation due to such a fixation is to convince people that there is no standard size, shape, consistency, or color. Sir Arthur Hurst indeed suggested that these people should be educated to the example of the dog rather than that of the cat, and never look behind them.

The people of the United States are said to spend more than $50 million a year to avoid constipation. Most of this is probably wasted, since it should be possible for practically every one to have a normal action of the bowel with proper habits of diet and bowel training.

Doctors know that the excessive use of cathartics tends to establish a habit which in the end damages the digestive tract. When the bowels get used to artificial stimulation, they are like a horse that will not run and requires more and more whipping as time goes on.

A good mixed diet with proper proteins, carbohydrates, fats, mineral salts, and vitamins and with enough indigestible residue is probably the most important single factor. People inclined toward delay in action of the bowel should take fruits, fresh or preserved, raw or cooked, with each meal and green vegetables or salad with both lunch and dinner. Stewed prunes for breakfast are considered particularly useful.

The various foods which contain amounts of bran are to be avoided, as they may irritate the bowel and they do not seem to have much advantage over fruits and vegetables. Indeed, foods with large quantities of bran should be considered medicinal foods and should be used only when prescribed by the doctor.

Among the drugs most commonly used to stir the

bowels to action are saline and vegetable cathartics, organic and mineral preparations, mechanically acting substances, and water in various forms. The continued use of strong salts may so irritate the lower portions of the bowel as to produce colitis. The vegetable cathartics like cascara, senna, aloes, rhubarb, and jalap act by irritating the bowel. Since irritation is abnormal, it is not well to make a habit of using any such cathartics.

The mechanically acting substances include mineral oil or liquid petrolatum, agar-agar (which is a seaweed), psyllium seeds, flax seeds, and bran. One of the chief arguments against the continued use of mineral oil is the fact that it absorbs vitamin A and may produce a vitamin A deficiency if used too constantly in connection with a deficient diet. Sometimes the use of mineral oil is unfortunate because of leakage of the material from the bowel. Mixtures of mineral oil with agar-agar or other substances, psyllium seeds and flax seeds develop a mucilaginous, bulky material useful in cases when failure of the bowel to act is the result of insufficient residue. In any event, it is necessary to know the nature of the constipation before determining which preparations are desirable in any specific case.

The majority of cases of dyschesia require re-education to get a good result, but in many such cases the first step is to develop a habit through the use of a mild enema or suppository. Just what is to be used in any given case should be determined by the doctor.

It is well established that regular exercise helps to keep the bowels active and is important particularly for people who are confined to a desk most of the day. For such people a five-minute walk before or after breakfast may be a good habit to establish.

Exercise of the abdominal muscles may be ordered when the failure of the bowel to act seems to be due to weakness of the muscles that are involved in the act of emptying the bowel.

People who are confined to bed and suffer from constipation may be helped by establishing a regular attempt to move the bowels immediately after breakfast. The toilet or commode should be used if possible. Some people find it difficult, if not actually impossible, to use a bedpan.

If three days have passed without a bowel movement, an enema may be given by the nurse or other attendant. In giving an enema, a bath mat is spread to avoid soiling of the floor. An enema bag containing a quart of lukewarm tapwater is hung not more than 2½–3 feet from the floor. The person may control the flow of water by pinching the tube. He lies on his left side and inserts the nozzle. Whenever pain is felt in the lower abdomen, the flow should be stopped until the pain disappears. In this manner as much as a quart of fluid can be introduced slowly.

People who are traveling can use some of the prepared enemas now available in the drugstores in plastic tubes.

Many physicians recommend that the person who is confined to bed and suffering from constipation take, two nights out of three, any of the common laxative preparations like milk of magnesia or cascara.

Nine
HEMORRHOIDS

Hemorrhoids are collections of varicose veins which are underneath the mucous membranes at the lower end of the bowel. Eighty per cent of people between thirty and sixty years old have them. Sometimes the person can feel them with the finger, but only the doctor who looks at them with an understanding eye can know exactly how minor or major they are. When they increase in size, when they protrude out of the bowel, when they become irritated or infected, they make their presence known.

Hemorrhoids have been described in the advertisements as itching, bleeding, and protruding. When they get bad enough, painful enough, or disturbing enough, they should be removed surgically because that is not too difficult an operation and brings complete relief. Many people prefer to try medical treatment before resorting to surgery. Small hemorrhoids that have not protruded can be injected with a coagulating solution which the doctor selects. Ultimately just a fibrous scar is left where the hemorrhoid was. Until the patient and the doctor have decided on the operation, temporizing is possible by the use of home care with materials that may be purchased in any drugstore.

Scrupulous cleanliness with soap and water will avert infection. However, use of strong soaps may irritate and induce infection. Resting off your feet will relieve pressure on varicose veins in the legs or in the rectum. The diet should be bland, avoiding nuts, corn, bran, seeds, strong condiments, and alcohol. Warm packs of gauze soaked in water that is hot but not burning may be applied three times a day for about an hour.

A wide variety of suppositories can be obtained without prescription and also ointments that come with the proper tube and nozzle for injection through the anus into the rectum. Some suppositories must be prescribed by the doctor because of the strength of the medicines they contain. Most of them have anti-itching and anesthetic substances designed to alleviate the pain, burning, and itching and to prevent destruction of tissue. They also contain mild antiseptics and astringents to constrict or shrink the blood vessels. For simple hemorrhoids, in order to reduce swelling, the doctor may wish to prescribe suppositories containing in addition to the usual softening and anesthetic substances some hydrocortisone, which is anti-inflammatory.

Ten
ANEMIA

The blood is the most important material of the body. Pumped by the heart, it carries all the nutriments and chemicals to the various tissues of the body and removes from these tissues the waste products that develop which are then excreted through the bowels, the kidneys, the sweat, and the exhaled air.

Blood is mostly water—about 55 per cent. The rest of it contains many chemicals which the doctor can determine by chemical examination. The solid or cellular elements of the blood are enormous numbers of little globules which are called red cells, white cells, and platelets. The cells are not manufactured in the blood but are developed by the millions in the marrow of the bones. When the cells are manufactured, they are discharged into the bloodstream where they function for a short period before they are replaced. The red cell is chiefly responsible for carrying in oxygen and carrying out carbon dioxide. A red cell is bright red when filled with oxygen. The blue color of a vein indicates that the red cells which it is carrying back to the lungs have given up their oxygen and are carrying carbon dioxide back to the lung spaces to be breathed out. Oxygen is picked up for use by the tissues.

In manufacturing red cells the bone marrow has to be supplied with the basic materials. These come chiefly from food. Some vitamins, copper, iron, and protein are needed. Iron is needed particularly for the manufacture of the hemoglobin or red coloring matter of the blood. The bone marrow properly supplied with these materials and performing its functions will produce trillions of blood cells every day.

A person with anemia has fewer red blood cells or less hemoglobin than needed to carry on the usual functions of the blood. Anemia is a symptom that something is wrong in the body. The exact cause has to be found in order to treat the anemia specifically. Anemia may be due either to a loss or to increased destruction of red blood cells. The loss may come through hemorrhage, which may be so gradual as to be unnoticed.

When a doctor wants to find out why a person is anemic, he makes a complete examination using laboratory tests, counting the various cells, and determining how much hemoglobin is present. The amount of yellowish pigment (called bilirubin) in the blood is a measure of the rate of blood-cell destruction.

Any severe anemia should be given prompt medical attention. However, mild degrees of anemia occur frequently because of inadequate building materials supplied to the bone marrow or because of the loss of blood from menstruation. Furthermore, some forms of anemia may result from the fact that the stomach is not able to absorb the iron needed because of a lack of hydrochloric acid secreted in the digestive juices of the stomach. In most cases of ordinary secondary anemia a deficiency of iron is discovered, and sometimes also a deficiency of certain vitamins.

Before 1926 every patient with pernicious anemia died. The cause of pernicious anemia is now known as a failure of the body to receive certain necessary substances or to absorb them or to make them available to the tissues. A specific substance for overcoming pernicious anemia has been found in the liver. More recently vitamin B_{12} was found to have the necessary properties for this purpose.

Women are especially vulnerable to anemias. When they begin to menstruate, they lose from two to five ounces of blood every month, and with the blood goes the iron that it carries. Every successive pregnancy cuts down the mother's store of iron. The growing baby abstracts from the blood of the mother the red coloring matter and other blood-building substances. Men who have frequent nosebleeds or who bleed from hemorrhoids or from some hidden cause in the stomach or bowels may also lose red coloring matter and iron.

Once the physician determines that anemia is due to some of these easily recognized causes, he will try to correct the cause and prescribe the materials necessary to substitute for what has been lost. The doctor treats iron-deficiency anemia by supplying iron. In unusual cases the iron may be given by injection, but in most instances it is taken in the form of tablets or solutions. At the same time the blood is studied at regular intervals to make sure that the iron is having the desired effect. An excess of iron may be harmful. However, the dosages printed on the labels of various preparations of iron in tablets, capsules, or solutions, which can be bought without a prescription, may be depended on as not likely to be harmful. If the recommended dosages are followed carefully, iron preparations are safe and reliable.

Eleven
FEVERS

Some doctors, particularly pediatricians, become exasperated because the mothers of their tiny patients are thermometer addicts. The minds of these mothers are fixed on the concept that a normal body temperature is near to 98.6° F. and that anything above or below that is a danger signal. Actually the body temperature varies depending on where the temperature is taken, the time of day, and the age of the patient. Temperature in the rectum or the vagina will be higher than when taken by mouth or under the arm. Physical exercise, a meal, emotional excitement, and menstruation also affect temperature.

Not everyone knows how to read a thermometer properly. At the beginning the thermometer should be shaken down until it reads below 95° F. Little children should have the temperature taken by rectum; when the child passes five or six years of age, it may be able to cooperate in taking temperature by mouth. Remember, never take the temperature just after a person has had a hot or cold drink. Many thermometers are marked to register in one-half minute, others for one minute. Probably it is best to leave them in the mouth double the time for which they are marked. Then take the thermometer out, read it, and put it back again to double-check.

Each time the thermometer is used it should be washed thoroughly with soap and water and dried with a clean paper napkin. Then shake down the mercury and put the thermometer back in its case. Always keep the thermometer in the same place so that time will not be lost looking for it when it is really needed.

When the temperature rises above ordinary limits— namely, 99° F.—the condition is called fever. Fever is an indication of illness, although not always an infectious disease or not even always an inflammation. Fever should be taken as a warning, just as pain is a warning.

If the fever is associated with chills, that is another reason for taking precautions. Probably the best thing to do is to get to bed and call the doctor. Long-continued fevers may burn important tissues of the body. Exercise or activity during a fever increases the fever. In children fevers below 100 degrees are not a cause for serious concern. If the person has chills he may be kept warm with blankets, by the application of hot-water bottles, or even by a tepid sponge bath.

Many superstitions prevail about fevers, such as "Feed a cold and starve a fever"; this has been proved to be without merit. If a person is hungry he can take food, which will give him calories to replace those burned by the fever. A sound rule is to give the fever patient plenty of fluids. If he sweats profusely for some time, the salt loss can be replaced by moderate amounts of salt added to the food and drink.

The medical profession used to rely heavily on drugs to ease fever; now lukewarm sponging may be tried. The drugs are called antipyretics. Aspirin is not only a reliever of pain but also an antipyretic. Unless the fever is exceedingly high, strong reducers are not tried.

Fevers appear frequently with coughs, colds, chills, infections of the nose, throat, and ear, and influenza. Fevers appear with infections within the body and accumulations of infectious material as in appendicitis, mastoiditis, infections in the internal ear, or even an abscess around a fingernail or toenail. In such instances, when the pus is removed, the fever will fall.

Twelve

OBESITY AND METERED FOODS

Back in the 1920's something called the eighteen-day Hollywood diet appeared in the United States and overnight the American public became calorie-conscious. A book called *Diet and Health with a Key to the Calories* sold millions of copies. Reports came from insurance companies that overweight after middle age was a hazard to health. Drugstores began displaying scales for daily weighing, foods to aid reduction of weight by helping to diminish calories, and substances called anorexiants, which reduce appetite. Eventually, rollers designed to roll off weight and innumerable devices to encourage muscular exercise arrived on the reducing scene.

The Anorexiants. Most of the substances now available for interfering with appetite are derivatives of benzedrine or amphetamine, which have the unfortunate duplicate effect of raising blood pressure and stimulating emotional reactions. Hence the length of time over which people may take these drugs is definitely limited. Preferably they are used in effective doses for a short time. More recently a new anorexiant has appeared which is without this stimulating effect but which occasionally in susceptible people may also have uncomfortable side effects.

Metered Foods. As an aid to dieting, many foods have appeared (largely in liquid form) which provide a limited number of calories—usually about nine hundred—together with protein, mineral salts, and vitamins. People on restricted diets often lack these essential substances. With the aid of a nine hundred-calorie diet designed to provide essential substances, a person can reduce weight, frequently as much as several pounds per week. However, liquid diets taken over too long a time eventually interfere with the action of the muscular tissue in the walls of the stomach and intestines. I once said that liquid diets are suitable to two periods in a person's life—first childhood and second childhood. To meet the objections against total liquid diets, some of the dietary foods have been prepared in the form of biscuits which contain enough cellulose or fibrous material to provide roughage without too many additional calories. Methyl cellulose is a nondigestible but otherwise harmless bulk material which helps to keep down the appetite by filling the stomach.

Necessary to weight reduction are will power and knowledge. Reduction of weight is a matter of physiological bookkeeping. You have to know how many calories there are in the quantities of foods you eat and you have to know how many calories you use up by your daily activities. About twelve hundred calories per day is called a basal requirement. Reduction of calories below twelve hundred will result in loss of weight. The rapidity of the loss of weight varies with the amount of reduction. Such starvation regimens as the eighteen-day Hollywood diet and other widely promoted diets have gone as low as six hundred calories a day.

Strict dieting should never be attempted without the advice of a competent physician or nutritionist. For one thing, obesity is often related to an emotional disturbance or to boredom or to some mental cause which must be controlled if dieting is to be effective.

There are also dietary foods for people who have to do without salt. These are salt substitutes. For people with diabetes, foods are available which are restricted in sugar content and which depend on the use of artificial sweeteners like Sucaryl® and Saccharine®. These artificial sweeteners are similarly helpful to those who have to cut down calories.

Thirteen
CARE OF THE FEET

When man assumed the erect posture he brought new stresses on the feet as well as the back. Anyone with a persistent pain in the feet needs an extensive examination by a competent orthopedic surgeon who, with the aid of X-ray pictures and other devices, will be able to determine whether or not the physical structure of the feet has in any way become abnormal.

Flat feet, which is usually a breaking down of the arch of the foot, used to be considered such a severe abnormality that men suffering from it were exempted from service with the Armed Forces. More recently the wide prevalence of flat feet has become recognized, and short of crippling cases, people with flat feet are not considered very abnormal.

Pain in the feet can also come from other causes. The pain may be associated with calluses on the bottom of the feet, corns, warts, and other changes in the tissues which irritate nerve endings. Some simple hints include an understanding of the fact that warm water will soften the skin and nails and permit easier removal of calluses, dead skin, or warts.

To prevent injury, the toenails should be cut straight across, using a scissors or nail clippers. If the nails are thickened or penetrate the tissue and cannot easily be cut with scissors, the person should have the attention of a competent podiatrist or chiropodist.

After bathing, the feet should be well dried, especially between the toes, and be powdered lightly with any good foot powder. If the skin is unusually dry, the skin of the feet like the skin of the face may be softened by using lanolin, baby oil, or any good foot cream. If the feet perspire greatly or tend to be irritated between the toes, some sterile cotton or lamb's wool may be kept between the toes.

In the drugstore one finds corn and callus removers which depend principally on preparations of salicylic acid to soften the tissue so that it may be removed. Corn plasters and corn pads work the same way. Some companies, like Scholl, have specialized in preparing all sorts of powders, sprays, and other materials for foot comfort. Among the leading foot powders are those of Scholl, Johnson & Johnson, and Mennen, but many of the leading drug companies also manufacture foot powders. The foot powder may contain a deodorant, a small dose of salicylate for softening tissue and preventing itching, and some preparations of hydroxyquinoline designed to act against ringworm.

Another group of products widely used for foot care are Desenex®. The base of most foot powders is talcum powder, but they may also include some boric acid and occasionally exceedingly small amounts of cooling preparations such as menthol. Some preparations designed particularly to control perspiration contain aluminum derivatives.

ATHLETE'S FOOT

Just about everyone who has ever walked barefoot has experienced an infection with the parasite that causes ringworm of the skin or athlete's foot. During the summer months specialists who take care of diseases of the skin see more athlete's foot than almost any other condition. It is the third most common skin disease in summer and the fifth in winter.

The germs that cause athlete's foot are generally known as fungi. There are many varieties of such fungi, and for a long time there were about as many methods of treatment. In recent years the causes have been more clearly defined, and more specific methods of treatment have been discovered.

Athlete's foot usually starts in the toenails, between the toes, or on the soles of the feet. The fungi can grow only in dead tissue. Therefore, they grow where there is an ample supply of dead, horny, or moist material such as is found on the soles of the feet and between the toes.

Care of the Feet

Most attacks occur in summer when people walk barefoot at swimming pools, in gymnasiums, or when they walk longer distances wearing shoes and socks that promote perspiration and moisture. Since the organisms or fungi are widespread, just about everyone has them constantly on the feet, around the toenails, in a small callus, in a soft corn, or in a fold of skin or a crack between the toes. Occasionally the infestation may spread to the hands from the feet or from the hands to the skin elsewhere on the body. The face and scalp are, however, seldom, if ever, affected.

Prevention

Dr. Marion Sulzberger has listed some simple ways to prevent athlete's foot:

1. Dry carefully and thoroughly the spaces between the toes, and in all other areas where skin folds are close together: groins, under breasts, under arms, and between buttocks.

2. Use a mild alcoholic solution—such as a 25 or 50 per cent rubbing alcohol, or a toilet water—on these areas after drying.

3. Liberally apply a plain, unscented talcum, or talcum and kaolin plus 5 per cent powdered boric acid to these areas and in socks, stockings, and shoes.

4. Treat all cracks or sogginess between the toes with an available antiseptic solution.

5. Remove crumbly nail material; keep the nails cut short.

6. Remove scaly, soggy, or excessively horny material from the soles of the feet.

7. Wear socks that are absorbent but not too coarse. Shoes should be well fitting but not too airtight; sufficiently roomy, but not large enough to chafe or rub.

8. Place pledgets of lamb's wool, absorbent cotton, or soft linen between toes that are too close together.

9. Consult a physician as soon as there is progressive redness, blistering, scaling, or itching which does not yield promptly to the measures described.

In addition, most experts recommend the following precautions:

1. Shoes or slippers should be worn at all times, especially when walking on wet floors or on wet ground.

2. Slippers, shoes, and socks should be kept dry and clean and replaced at suitable intervals. They should never be worn by other persons whose feet may be infected with fungi.

3. Bathtubs, bathmats, and floors in households in which a member is suffering from athlete's foot should be sponged or cleansed regularly with hot water and soap.

4. After visits to public beaches, pools, etc., uninfected people should apply to their feet preparations designed to kill fungi—for example, 1 part full strength tincture of iodine diluted with 10 parts of alcohol, or

a 1 per cent solution of gentian violet, or one of the newly available preparations containing undecylenic acid or propionic acid.

5. An infected member of a household should, when possible, be given either a separate bathroom, or a separate bathmat, towel, etc. Persons known to be infected should not be permitted to come into intimate physical contact with other, noninfected members of the family.

If your feet are infected, keep your shoes off as much as possible and stay off your feet. When the skin becomes swollen, blistered, red, or itching, doctors prescribe compresses soaked in a solution called Burrow's solution or a solution of aluminum subacetate. The blisters may be opened with a sterilized pin or needle, preferably sterilized by passing through a flame. The cracks and the bases of the blisters may be treated with an available antiseptic solution. At night a calomine lotion, either plain or with 1 per cent of menthol, may be applied to stop the itching. After healing, pastes of zinc oxide or zinc-oxide ointment may be used. White cotton socks may be worn in bed to keep the ointment in contact with the skin at night.

Among recent discoveries has been the knowledge that powders or ointments which contain propionate or undecylenic acid may be specifically helpful against athlete's foot either for curing it or for maintaining the resistance to infestation. Such powders are now available without prescription in many forms. Some which include preparations of cortisone or other agents must be prescribed by the doctor. Recently also certain antibiotics have been discovered capable of acting specifically against fungi. These are derivatives of griseofulvin and must be prescribed by the doctor. When this substance is taken internally, it develops resistance against the fungi.

Fourteen
FEMININE HYGIENE

Menstruation has tended to move away from consideration as a normal physiologic process into a belief that all sorts of special cleansing techniques are required for hygienic purposes. The drugstores make available a great variety of products designed for this purpose, including many that are to be had only on prescription by the physician. Any real disturbance of menstruation, such as irregularity, extraordinary pain, accumulation of fluid, headache, or swelling, should have the attention of a physician.

Disagreeable odor is in many instances associated with infections which may involve a wide variety of germs. Necessary is a determination of the nature of the infection in order to provide the most effective treatment. Among the most frequent of infections associated with severe odors is a condition called trichomoniasis, which is controlled successfully by a special antibiotic in most instances. This is called Flagyl® or Metronidazole,

97

which must also be prescribed by a physician. Otherwise treatment in the past was dependent on douching with various antiseptic preparations which, however, were not especially effective.

Dysmenorrhea, or painful menstruation, is associated with overtiredness, constipation, and sometimes exceptional sensitivity to pain. Remedies similar to those used for headache or other pains are frequently taken at this time.

Excessive bleeding should always be reported to a physician. Sometimes anemia results, requiring appropriate treatment. Irregularities of menstruation must be studied by the physician. Sometimes treatment is possible with hormones.

A discharge between menstruations or pain in the genital organs in adult women may be associated with inadequate hygiene. Some women have not learned that cleansing of the region between the anus and the genitals and, in fact, wiping of the genitals should always be from the front toward the back to avoid possibility of infection from the excretions.

The pharmacies supply preparations which under our food and drug laws are well controlled as to safety. These include sanitary napkins and tampons as well as special douches, disinfectants, and vaginal foams. In general, women in good health who observe ordinary hygiene will not require frequent and daily douching. If, however, any of the symptoms mentioned appear, the physician may well prescribe what he thinks is desirable, and instruct as to frequency and methods of use.

Fifteen
VITAMINS

The main constituents of food are proteins, carbohydrates, fats, mineral salts, and vitamins. To many people the vitamins are just letters in the alphabet from A to E with several parts of B and some K and P, about which there are still some doubts. Actually vitamins are chemical substances whose importance is recognized more by what happens when they are absent than by the positive effects occasioned by their presence. Their presence in the diet may mean the difference between abundant health and just ordinary vitality.

Only about half a century has passed since the word "vitamin" came into our vocabulary. The term was invented by a Pole named Casimir Funk, working in London during the years just before the First World War. It was combined from two terms—the first meaning life, and the second referring to a chemical substance. Today it is known that the vitamins are not "amins" but they are, of course, necessary to life.

In the eighteenth century British sailors found out that

something in the diet was necessary to prevent scurvy. Dr. James Lind discovered what the something was—a sufficient amount of fresh fruit and vegetables.

Around 1826 a French physiologist, François Magendie, found that dogs fed on fine white bread and water died after fifty days, but dogs fed on coarse miliary bread (ground from millet) lived and kept their health. Toward the end of the nineteenth century Christiaan Eijkman, a Dutch doctor in Java, discovered that people who ate polished rice developed a form of paralysis and inflammation of the nerves, but that those eating the whole rice did not develop these symptoms. Even chickens which ate polished rice developed the disease. Experimentally he proved the possibility of producing beriberi, which is the form of neuritis resulting from a lack of vitamin B in the diet, by feeding a diet free from vitamin B, and he was rewarded for his investigations by the Nobel Prize in 1929.

Since 1910 vitamin research has developed at a tremendous rate. Books are available in profusion, and vitamin products pack the shelves of the drugstores and the groceries. It may seem strange that little or nothing was heard of the vitamins in all the earlier years of man's existence on this earth, yet it is not strange if one pauses to consider how our civilization has changed during the last century. In an earlier day people lived outdoors much more than now and obtained plenty of sunlight. Before the sophistication of food was begun people ate what came directly from the farm or from animal sources with-

out much modification. When men began to crowd together in great cities and to catch diseases freely, when
it became necessary to ship foods over long distances
and to preserve them for long periods to satisfy the needs
of the city dwellers, the food substances began to be
changed.

Boiling food destroys some vitamins, and oxidation
destroys others. Chemical processes may remove all
vitamins from certain foods. Some vitamins deteriorate
when the foods are preserved for long periods; it may not
be taken for granted that the food as served on the table
contains the vitamins that were in it when it left the farm.

Certain foods contain certain vitamins in large
amounts, others in lesser amounts, and still others not
at all. One must be properly informed if one is to have all
of the vitamins one needs for healthy growth and prevention of disease. Yet the information need not be de-
tailed or exact if one eats a wide variety of food
substances and makes certain that some of these are in
the raw or natural state.

The fact is now well established that certain vitamins
are necessary to suitable growth of the animal body. In
their absence the body becomes stunted and the tissues
weak. A complete deficiency of any one of the vitamins
will inevitably result in the appearance of disease and
of degeneration of the tissues, and partial absence of the
vitamins will result in symptoms which indicate ineffi-
ciency of the tissues.

Vitamins A and D are fat-soluble vitamins and are discussed together. The other vitamins are water soluble.

VITAMIN A

Most vitamin A needed by the human body can be readily acquired by choosing the right foods. Vitamin A is found in rather large amounts in milk, butter, eggs, cod liver oil, halibut liver oil, carrots, the green leafy vegetables, and as an added substance in modern commercial margarine. Scientists have found that summer milk may contain twice as much vitamin A as does winter milk. Vitamin A content of ordinary cow's milk depends on the diet of the cow. Human milk usually contains more vitamin A than cow's milk, but this also is dependent on the diet of the mother.

About 90 per cent of the vitamin A in the human body is stored in the liver. If no additional vitamin A is taken into the body, the absence will not be noted for three months to a year or more. Some vitamin A is found in the blood.

When there is a lack of vitamin A it is usually due to lack of carotin, which is the precursor of vitamin A in the diet. However, because of various conditions there may be interference with absorption or storage of vitamin A, interference with the conversion of carotin to vitamin A, or a rapid loss of vitamin A from the body. Deficiency of this vitamin may accompany such diseases as sprue, cystic fibrosis of the pancreas, and ulcerative colitis. It may be a factor in complications following some surgical operations, in obstruction of the bowel, and cirrhosis of the liver. In diabetes and in hypothyroidism, the body may fail to convert carotin into vitamin A. Also there is some loss of vitamin A in various infectious diseases of childhood. Sometimes when a child is sensitive to milk and soybean milk is substituted for cow's milk, a vitamin A deficiency may result. Hence such infants are given extra vitamin A.

The chief condition resulting from a deficiency of vitamin A is night blindness, followed by inflammation of the eye, sometimes resulting in total blindness. In severe malnutrition resulting from a lack of vitamin A a condition called xerophthalmia occurs with dryness of the cornea (the membrane on the front of the eye) which may result in total blindness. Dryness, roughness, and wrinkling of the conjunctiva are followed by swelling and redness of the lids, pain (particularly in bright light). In such cases adequate feeding of vitamin A can cure the condition.

Old people sometimes suffer from a lack of vitamin A because of inadequate diet or inability to convert carotin into vitamin A. Other experiments have shown that the skin and all epithelial tissues must have adequate vitamin A or they tend to hardening and inadequate function. Epithelial tissues include not only the skin but the lining of the respiratory, gastrointestinal, and genitourinary tracts, also the salivary glands, the glands of internal secretion, and the vagina. For these reasons many specialists in conditions affecting the skin prescribe vitamin A as a part of their treatment for various skin conditions associated with dryness of the skin and the scalp.

The average healthy person does not need any supplement of vitamin A provided he is eating an adequate diet. However, many people, including the ill, the overweight, and those who suffer from a variety of digestive disturbances are not likely to have a completely adequate diet. For such people supplementary vitamin A is desirable, taken either as the vitamin A in tablets alone or in combination with other needed vitamins. In cases of severe deprivation, when large doses of vitamin A may be necessary, the physician may prescribe a variety of forms, in very large doses, available in the drugstore.

VITAMIN D

Vitamin D is commonly called the sunshine vitamin. The beneficial effects of sunshine were observed long before vitamin D was related to the sun's rays. The children of the poor living in crowded slums frequently developed rickets. Once in England a tax was placed on windows, and industrial buildings began to reduce the number of windows. Rickets became so common that it was called the English disease. From 1645 onward medical speculation was rife. Various mineral salts, calcium, and phosphorus were erroneously alleged to be the missing substances in the diets of rachitics. In 1890 a doctor practicing in Japan was struck by the absence of rickets in that country. He saw that cold and wet climate and lack of sunlight were in some way related to rickets. His actual words were, "Sunlight is essential to the healthy nutrition of growing animals and a deficiency of it characterizes the localities and conditions of those who suffer from rickets and is the most important element in the etiology of that disease."

Today we know that vitamin D is necessary to permit the body to use calcium and phosphorus for the formation of sound bones and teeth. This is particularly important with growing children. Vitamin D is also associated in some way with the use of citric acid by the body.

Among newborn infants without any supplementary vitamin D, the calcium is deficient in about 16 per cent. To assure a vitamin D sufficiency, cod liver oil and other sources have long been available. In recent times large doses of vitamin D have been given in all sorts of conditions where calcium may be involved. Tremendous doses of vitamin D are dangerous, as are excessive doses of vitamin A. Such large doses involve deposits of calcium in vital organs which may be exceedingly harmful.

The only way a mother can calculate the amount of vitamin D in her child's food is to ascertain the value of all the child's food in terms of substances providing vitamin D. Of course one may also obtain some of the effects of vitamin D by exposure to natural sunlight or to ultraviolet rays. However, overexposure to the sun is a menace to health; overexposure to ultraviolet rays may produce severe burns. Nowadays many safer means have been found for giving vitamin D in addition to the use of cod liver and halibut liver oils or condensates of such oils. A cow fed irradiated yeast will give milk rich in vitamin D, or the milk itself may be irradiated with the same effect. Vitamin D is also available in mixtures of vitamins such as a great variety of tablets made by many manufacturers which are available in drugstores.

Most dietetic authorities are convinced that the American diet contains insufficient amounts of calcium. At the same time city smog screens out much sunlight. Most infants and growing children, therefore, who live in cities can use some extra vitamins A and D. But the adult whose bones and teeth have developed fully will gain little, if anything, by taking extra vitamin D.

VITAMIN C

The chemical name for vitamin C is ascorbic acid. This name refers to the fact that vitamin C is a preventive of scurvy and, therefore, an antiscorbutic substance. Scurvy, a disease which appears when there is a lack of vitamin C in the body either because of insufficient intake or because the body cannot use what is taken in, has been known since at least 1500 B.C. Yet only in recent years has it been fully controllable. As early as 1906, before the word vitamin was invented, a scientist suggested that infantile scurvy was a deficiency disease.

Among foods rich in vitamin C are all the citrus fruits (oranges, lemons, grapefruit, limes, and tangerines), but also most of the fruits and the green vegetables. Usually vitamin C content is measured in milligrams of ascorbic acid per 100 grams of the food. Especially interesting, therefore, is the fact that raw broccoli has a rating of 118, raw collards 100, guavas 302, parsley 193, and turnip greens 136, compared with 49 for oranges. However, cooking results in the loss of much vitamin C. Whereas raw broccoli has a rating of 118, cooked broccoli has a rating of 74. Turnip greens raw rate 136, but cooked turnip greens drop to 60.

In general, meats, cereals, and dairy products contain such small amounts of vitamin C as to be unimportant in this connection. In addition to the citrus fruits, tomatoes and tomato juice are mentioned particularly. More recently nutritionists have reported that the juice of the Puerto Rican wild cherry has been found to be eighty times as rich in vitamin C as orange juice; it has been marketed under the trademark name of Acerola®.

A peculiarity about vitamin C is that it is not retained in the body but used up rapidly. The National Research Council through its Food and Nutrition Board says that good nutrition can be maintained by an intake of from seventy to eighty milligrams of ascorbic acid daily. The proper amount for infants up to one year is thirty, that for growing children and teenagers sixty or seventy.

Research has shown many, many uses for vitamin C in the body in relationship not only to scurvy, which in its fullest manifestations is associated with failures of growth, hemorrhages, breakdown of the capillary blood vessels, and many other symptoms, but also in what might be called subacute vitamin C deficiency. The condition is detected by laboratory examinations.

When vitamin C is needed because of clearly apparent symptoms, the doctor will prescribe the substance as a drug. However, vitamin C is included in all multivitamin tablets in adequate amounts. With the new knowledge of the usefulness of vitamin C, scurvy has just about disappeared in the United States. All mothers are instructed in the provision of orange juice and other good sources of vitamin C. It is worth mentioning here, however, that tomato juice is only about half as rich as orange juice, while pineapple juice, despite its pleasant flavor, is not a good source at all.

VITAMIN B

Vitamin B has now been determined to contain many substances of the greatest importance to human health and growth. Therefore, one usually speaks of it as the vitamin B complex. In it are included thiamine (formerly known as vitamin B_1), riboflavin, niacin, pyridoxine (formerly called vitamin B_6), folic acid, vitamin B_{12}, which is a life-saving product in pernicious anemia, biotin, and pantothenic acid.

Beriberi, of which the chief manifestation is peripheral neuritis, was once as widespread as an epidemic. It developed because primitive groups ate polished rice, losing the advantage of the thiamine contained in the hull. Used as a drug, thiamine is prescribed in a variety of conditions related to accumulation of water in some portion of the body and in various forms of neuritis. However, lack of thiamine is related to the appearance in the human tissue of pyruvic acid and, therefore, of symptoms resulting from the effects of that substance. Thiamine deficiency is noted particularly in people who are chronic alcoholics, and the symptoms affect the eyes, the nerves, and the brain.

The richest sources of thiamine are pork, liver, yeast, whole cereals, and fresh green vegetables. Milk, which may be called the most nearly perfect food, does not provide adequate thiamine. People on restricted diets must, therefore, get thiamine prescribed by the doctor. The Food and Nutrition Board has calculated thiamine requirements at 0.4 milligrams of thiamine for every thousand calories of food. Extra thiamine is needed during pregnancy and particularly for nursing mothers. Thiamine is also a constituent of practically all multivitamin tablets.

Riboflavin. A real deficiency of riboflavin in the diet will be manifested by inflammations around the mouth, seborrheic dermatitis particularly around the nose, and changes in the eyes. Again, restricted diets with insufficient amounts of animal food and dairy proteins will produce some of the symptoms of riboflavin deficiency. Overcooking of vegetables or other foods results in destruction of riboflavin. The substance is available for prescription by the doctor in true cases of riboflavin deficiency, and it is included in all multivitamin tablets.

Nicotinic Acid. The vital importance of nicotinic acid was proved when investigators found that pellagra, which once affected hundreds of thousands of people in the United States, was due to a lack of this vitamin. A condition called black tongue in dogs was proved to be a deficiency disease related to absence of nicotinic acid. This substance takes part in many of the important functions of the body due to the part it plays in some of the chemical reactions.

A real deficiency of nicotinic acid is shown by such symptoms as weakness, lassitude, loss of appetite, and indigestion, followed, as in the case of pellagra, by dermatitis, diarrhea, and dementia. The dermatitis appears particularly in the parts of the body exposed to sunlight and heat.

When the intake of nicotinic acid is less than 715 milligrams a day, pellagra may appear. Hence the drug is included in all multivitamin formulas in amounts related to the essential requirements. The amounts usually included in all such tablets is ten milligrams. Its purpose is to meet any vitamin deficiency, but it is especially important in pregnancy, in wasting diseases, in restricted diets, or in instances when the body apparently is unable to absorb and utilize the nicotinic acid found in ordinary foods.

Pantothenic Acid. Pantothenic acid is another portion of the vitamin B complex which is frequently included in multivitamin tablets. In some animals, notably chicks and rats, it has specific functions related to the skin. It had been exploited at one time as of special value in preventing gray hair, because rats with an insufficient amount of it develop gray hair. However, there is so much pantothenic acid in so many common foods that a deficiency of this vitamin is very unusual. Some scientific investigators have reported that pantothenic acid gave relief in certain disturbances of the nervous system and in burning of the skin. However, this is empirical since there has been no proof that there is a deficiency of pantothenic acid in such cases. If, however, people are intentionally deprived of all pantothenic acid in the diet and are given a substance which acts against pantothenic acid, they will develop many different symptoms, including muscle cramps and impaired coordination.

Obviously pantothenic acid has a most important role in human nutrition. Doubtful, however, is the possibility that real pantothenic-acid deficiency occurs except under most extraordinary circumstances, such as gross malnutrition.

Pyridoxine. Several portions of the vitamin B complex are classified as the vitamin B$_6$ group, which are mostly pyridoxines. Vitamin B$_6$ also occurs in many animal products and also in vegetables. It is plentiful in cow's milk, in lamb, pork, in wheat germ, and in soybean flour, for example. Large amounts are found in split peas, peanuts, and smaller amounts in whole wheat and rye bread.

Pyridoxine plays an important role in many chemical changes that go on in the body. There is still considerable mystery attached to its function. A deficiency of it brings on inflammations and disturbances of the skin. Not long ago infants who were being fed principally on a baby food that did not contain pyridoxine developed a convulsive disorder. When pyridoxine was added, the convulsions disappeared. Obstetricians have been using pyridoxine to control the nausea of pregnancy. This was done on the evidence that pyridoxine used by the body may be altered during pregnancy, so that more is needed.

People who are taking certain drugs such as isonicotinic acid, Hydrozid, or some of the anti-hypertensive products like Hydralazine, have developed nervous manifestations which come because these products interfere with the use by the body of pyridoxine.

In all such cases as those that have been described, extra pyridoxine may be given. The average diet in America provides more than enough pyridoxine, but restricted diets do not. Therefore pyridoxine is also a constituent of most multivitamin preparations.

Folic Acid. Included in the vitamin B complex is folic acid, which is found in considerable amounts in many foods and which is related to the development of blood cells and the red coloring matter of the blood. In the condition called pernicious anemia apparently the use of folic acid in the body is blocked in some way. Many people who have conditions like sprue and absorb folic acid poorly have low levels of folic acid in the blood and suffer with anemia-like conditions.

In animal nutrition folic acid is important for the action of many hormones.

Formerly folic acid was given to patients with pernicious anemia and seemed to substitute satisfactorily for the effects they got from liver and liver extracts. When folic acid was given to a patient with this disease, he began to create new blood cells on the third day, with the maximum rise by the eighth or tenth day. But more recently vitamin B_{12} has been used for such patients because patients on folic acid tended to develop nervous manifestations. These do not appear when vitamin B_{12} is given.

For a while folic acid was included in most multivitamin capsules, but more recently the product is used to treat more specific forms of anemia such as that which occurs in pregnancy or certain disorders in infants.

Vitamin B_{12}. The technical name for vitamin B_{12} is cobalamine. This vitamin is found almost exclusively in foods of animal origin, and is synthesized in the body by various bacteria. The best sources of vitamin B_{12} are liver, kidney, meat, and milk, with diminishing amounts in such foods as cheese, salmon, and oysters.

For proper absorption of vitamin B_{12} another factor found in the walls of the stomach is necessary. This vitamin has now been related to many of the basic chemical reactions that go on in the body and are necessary for health and life. Many conditions related to the stomach have been associated with a deficiency of vitamin B_{12}.

Combined deficiencies of vitamin B_{12} and folic acid in human diets bring on anemias. Therefore this vitamin is included in most multivitamin preparations and in certain severe forms of anemia is prescribed by doctors in specific amounts, even by injection. The vitamin has also been used in several forms of neuritis.

Bioflavonoids. In searching for new vitamins, a family of substances which resemble vitamins has been found. Sometimes these are called collectively vitamin P, although scientists prefer to call them bioflavonoids. Their absence from the diet has been associated with disturbances of the capillaries, with the appearance of blood spots on the skin, particularly in diabetes. Other chemical substances like choline, biotin, and inositol have been included in the B complex.

Certainly a severe deficiency of some of these substances may be associated with symptoms, but the exact relationships to health have not been sufficiently determined to make it seem reasonable that they be included even in multivitamin tablets, capsules, and mixtures.

VITAMIN K

A vitamin deficiency which results in hemorrhagic disease in chickens was found to be related to a substance found principally in the leafy vegetables and in alfalfa, which has been designated vitamin K. An adequate supply of bile salts is necessary for absorption of this vitamin in the intestines. A deficiency of vitamin K results in absence from the blood of a substance called prothrombin, which is important in coagulation of the blood.

Sometimes a deficiency is found in newborn infants. This usually disappears as the baby grows older. However, in some instances physicians supply extra vitamin K to overcome the deficiency and prevent unusual bleeding. When the liver is severely damaged by any kind of disease, the prothrombin concentration of the blood may be lowered.

This vitamin participates frequently in the oxidation and reduction of oxygen that take place in the body.

Occasionally this vitamin is also included in vitamin combinations.

VITAMIN E

For more than forty years vitamin E has been known to be necessary for reproduction in the rat. However, this vitamin has not been proved essential to human reproduction. Because of its effect on animals all sorts of studies have been made of the possible effects of deficiency of vitamin E in human beings, particularly in such conditions as pseudohypertrophic muscular dystrophy, habitual abortion, and, more recently, in coronary heart disease.

Notwithstanding a great deal of research, there seems to be no good reason why this vitamin should be included even in multivitamin tablets. People who eat vegetable oils, such as those obtained from corn, peanuts, soybeans, coconut, or cottonseed, people who eat cereal products and eggs are likely to get all the vitamin E they need and can use.

Sixteen

NAUSEA, DIZZINESS, MOTION SICKNESS, ANTACIDS, AND STOMACH SWEETENERS

Almost every family has a member who gets sick riding in an automobile, train, ship, or airplane. Motion sickness is usually associated with the action of the labyrinth in the inner ear. Sudden changes of direction and particularly rhythmical changes of direction affect the inner ear and the organs of balance. Pregnant women, children, and dogs are particularly susceptible.

Psychosomatic influence may have some responsibility in motion sickness. Many a young woman gets sick if she has to ride in the back seat but feels fine in the front. Perhaps such women suffer from some relationship between the sense of vision and the internal ear. This fits in with the observation that the driver of a car seldom gets carsick.

The early warning signs of beginning motion sickness include yawning, deep breathing, swallowing, after which comes a dry mouth and vomiting. A worthwhile precaution for people who easily get carsick or suffer from other symptoms of motion sickness is to avoid eating before traveling.

The law now permits the sale over the counter in drugstores of a variety of drugs which can prevent motion sickness. Among these the best known are Dramamine®, Bonamine®, and Marezine®. One dose should be taken about half an hour before starting on a journey. A second may be taken when the journey begins. Additional dosage may be required if symptoms develop. However, the limits beyond which one should not go in use of such anti-motion-sickness remedies are stated on the label and should be strictly observed.

ANTACIDS AND
STOMACH SWEETENERS

Judging from the shelves of our pharmacies, Americans take more pills, capsules, and solutions to correct what they assume to be difficulties with the acid in the stomach than any other people in the world.

The stomach, functioning normally, produces pepsin and hydrochloric acid. The hydrochloric acid serves many useful purposes. However, in cases of peptic ulcer, inflammation of the stomach, and hiatus or diaphragmatic hernia, doctors have found that lowering the acidity is helpful in relieving pain. If the acid content is too greatly reduced, the stomach will empty more rapidly, which will clear the drug out and end its useful effect.

Most antacids contain compounds of aluminum hydroxide, magnesium hydroxide, and calcium carbonate.

Some people suffer after eating from a sense of overfilling the stomach. In most cases this is due to swallowing air. Any mild alkaline substance or antacid will help to relieve this sensation. Antacids with sodium bicarbonate act by adding more gas, which causes the person to belch.

Keep in mind that the antacids do not stop the secretion of the acid in the stomach. They temporarily neutralize it. Since the acid continues to be secreted by the wall of the stomach, one dose of any antacid will not cure the basic condition. These drugs must be taken frequently. In peptic ulcer the doctor often directs the taking of milk or mixtures of milk and cream at fairly frequent intervals, alternating with doses of the antacid substance.

The victim of these conditions is primarily concerned with the pain, while the doctor is primarily concerned with healing the area in the stomach which causes the pain. In most cases he will recommend continuing the antacids even after the pain has largely disappeared, until sufficient protection has been given to permit healing of the injured area.

Some drugs are available which actually diminish the secretion of gastric juice. But these drugs can be taken only when prescribed by the doctor.

Seventeen
OINTMENTS, LINIMENTS, AND OTHER EXTERNAL MEDICATION

Everybody has troubles with the skin. Indeed, minor troubles are so frequent that sufficient doctors would never be available to look at all of them. It is hardly surprising that the shelves of a modern drugstore contain a wide variety of ointments, liniments, and lotions as well as many other preparations designed for use on the surface of the body. The restrictions under the Food and Drug Act on drugs to be applied externally are not so severe as those concerned with drugs taken internally. Apparently some people do not use the preparations wisely, because dermatologists insist that more patients come to them suffering from overtreatment applied by themselves than from almost any other cause.

A considerable number of athlete's foot remedies are also offered as antiseptics. Ointments containing camphor or menthol are designed to slightly irritate the skin, producing a moderate inflammation which is said to be helpful for a wide variety of pains and minor disorders.

Preparations which have been used over the years are helpful for chapping and chilblains. Mild preparations, which usually contain sulphur, are said to be helpful in acne and blackheads. Because pregnant women experience stretching of the skin which leaves marks after childbirth, there are preparations which are claimed to be useful in softening the skin and preventing permanent marking.

Psoriasis. Among the most troublesome of all skin diseases is psoriasis, for which a definite cause is not yet known and for which there is no specific method of treatment. Nevertheless, preparations are on the shelves for self-treatment of psoriasis, most of which are designed simply to prevent secondary infection and to lessen the scaling.

Burns. Since burns are common accidents, a considerable number of preparations are designed to lessen the pain of burns by covering the exposed area.

Sweating. Excessive sweat is a nuisance. Furthermore, germs multiply rapidly in the presence of warmth and wetness. When germs get into sweaty areas, inevitably an odor develops.

Many modern deodorants contain the mild antiseptic hexachlorophene which helps to keep off the germs, and various aluminum salt preparations which by their astringency prevent perspiration. The first step is probably washing with plenty of good soap and water. Then any of the antiperspirant and deodorant preparations can be applied. Experience will tell which is most helpful.

The advertising claims vary principally in respect to the way in which the preparation is used—whether sprayed on, rolled on, dabbed on, or some other way. One works about as well as another, depending on the user's preference.

Warts. Warts are a constant object of study by doctors. Viruses have been definitely associated with some types of warts. A recent study compared twenty-four boys whose warts were treated by various techniques with twenty-four boys in another group whose warts were left alone. After several years the boys who received treatment had just about the same number of new warts as the boys who did not.

Warts, however, are unsightly and may become irritated by the ordinary contacts of life. One method of treatment is simply to cover them with adhesive plaster. Cleverly contrived forms of bandages are now available.

The wart treatments on the drugstore shelves contain certain mild antiseptic remedies which may or may not help. In any case do not try to cut out a wart yourself and do not apply caustic substances like trichlorocetic acid. Such harsh measures are to be left to the doctor.

Sun-tanning. From a scientific point of view suntan is not particularly a sign of health. Tanning may well be a sign of overexposure to the sun. In response to the sun's rays, the body produces a pigment substance which is called melanin and which is deposited in the skin, acting as a filter to the ultraviolet rays of the sun. The dark-skinned races have natural protection against sunburn;

the lighter-skinned races burn more easily; fair-skinned and red-haired people are most easily burned.

Doctors have always recommended that exposure to the sun be gradual—a few minutes the first day, slowly increasing until the skin is sufficiently tanned to afford protection. However, the average vacation of a week or two in a sunny place hardly permits this kind of gradual suntan, and most teenagers as well as young adults like to prove that they had a good vacation by coming home with a nice suntan.

The modern suntan lotion contains drugs which help to screen out the ultraviolet rays that cause the burning. These suntan mixtures come as lotions, oils, creams, and recently sprays. Since these cosmetic preparations are controlled as to their content by the Food and Drug Administration, practically all of those commonly sold are safe and dependable if used according to the directions.

INSECT REPELLENTS
AND INSECTICIDES

The human being's usual response to the presence of insects is to try to get rid of them. The drugstore offers many repellents and insecticides, some of which are designed to repel the insects by their odors, others by destroying the insects or the places in which the insects live and breed. Any preparation capable of destroying insects can also make human beings sick if present in too large amounts, particularly in enclosed rooms. Such preparations should always be kept away from the eyes and the lips. And, once more, it is of cardinal importance to read the labels.

INDEX

Index

Index